Osteotomies Around the Knee

Editors

ANNUNZIATO (NED) AMENDOLA
DAVIDE EDOARDO BONASIA

CLINICS IN SPORTS MEDICINE

www.sportsmed.theclinics.com

Consulting Editor
MARK D. MILLER

July 2019 • Volume 38 • Number 3

ELSEVIER

1600 John F. Kennedy Boulevard • Suite 1800 • Philadelphia, Pennsylvania, 19103-2899

http://www.theclinics.com

CLINICS IN SPORTS MEDICINE Volume 38, Number 3
July 2019 ISSN 0278-5919, ISBN-13: 978-0-323-68207-7

Editor: Lauren Boyle
Developmental Editor: Donald Mumford

Clinics in Sports Medicine (ISSN 0278-5919) is published quarterly by Elsevier Inc., 360 Park Avenue South, New York, NY 10010-1710. Months of issue are January, April, July, and October. Business and Editorial Offices: 1600 John F. Kennedy Blvd., Ste. 1800, Philadelphia, PA 19103-2899. Customer Service Office: 3251 Riverport Lane, Maryland Heights, MO 63043. Periodicals postage paid at New York, NY and additional mailing offices. Subscription prices are $364.00 per year (US individuals), $698.00 per year (US institutions), $100.00 per year (US students), $405.00 per year (Canadian individuals), $861.00 per year (Canadian institutions), $235.00 (Canadian students), $475.00 per year (foreign individuals), $861.00 per year (foreign institutions), and $235.00 per year (foreign students). Foreign air speed delivery is included in all *Clinics* subscription prices. All prices are subject to change without notice. **POSTMASTER:** Send address changes to *Clinics in Sports Medicine*, Elsevier Health Sciences Division, Subscription Customer Service, 3251 Riverport Lane, Maryland Heights, MO 63043. Customer Service (orders, claims, online, change of address): Elsevier Health Sciences Division, Subscription Customer Service, 3251 Riverport Lane, Maryland Heights, MO 63043. **Tel: 1-800-654-2452 (U.S. and Canada); 314-447-8871 (outside U.S. and Canada). Fax: 314-447-8029. E-mail: journalscustomerservice-usa@elsevier.com (for print support); journalsonlinesupport-usa@elsevier.com (for online support).**

Reprints. For copies of 100 or more of articles in this publication, please contact the Commercial Reprints Department, Elsevier Inc., 360 Park Avenue South, New York, NY 10010-1710. Tel.: 212-633-3874; Fax: 212-633-3820; E-mail: reprints@elsevier.com

Clinics in Sports Medicine is covered in *MEDLINE/PubMed (Index Medicus) Current Contents/Clinical Medicine, Excerpta Medica,* and *ISI/Biomed.*

Contributors

CONSULTING EDITOR

MARK D. MILLER, MD
S. Ward Casscells Professor, Head, Department of Orthopaedic Surgery, Division of Sports Medicine, University of Virginia, Charlottesville, Virginia, USA; Team Physician, Miller Review Course, Harrisonburg, Virginia, USA

EDITORS

ANNUNZIATO (NED) AMENDOLA, MD
Director of Sports Medicine, Urbaniak Sports Sciences Institute, Duke University, Durham, North Carolina, USA

DAVIDE EDOARDO BONASIA, MD
Department of Orthopaedics and Traumatology, AO Ordine Mauriziano Hospital, University of Torino, Torino, Italy

AUTHORS

AVINESH AGARWALLA, MD
Department of Orthopaedic Surgery, Westchester Medical Center, Valhalla, New York, USA

C. THOMAS APPLETON, MD, PhD
Bone and Joint Institute, London Health Sciences Centre, University Hospital, Department of Physiology and Pharmacology, Schulich School of Medicine and Dentistry, Western University, London, Ontario, Canada

HAYDEN F. ATKINSON, BSc
Wolf Orthopaedic Biomechanics Laboratory, Fowler Kennedy Sport Medicine Clinic, Bone and Joint Institute, London Health Sciences Centre, University Hospital, School of Physical Therapy, Faculty of Health Sciences, Western University, London, Ontario, Canada

CHRISTOPHER D. BERNARD, BS
Department of Orthopedic Surgery and Sports Medicine, Mayo Clinic, Rochester, Minnesota, USA

TREVOR B. BIRMINGHAM, PT, PhD
Wolf Orthopaedic Biomechanics Laboratory, Fowler Kennedy Sport Medicine Clinic, Bone and Joint Institute, London Health Sciences Centre, University Hospital, School of Physical Therapy, Faculty of Health Sciences, Western University, London, Ontario, Canada

DAVIDE EDOARDO BONASIA, MD
Department of Orthopaedics and Traumatology, AO Ordine Mauriziano Hospital, University of Torino, Torino, Italy

LAURA BRAGONZONI, PhD
Laboratorio di Biomeccanica e Innovazione Tecnologica, Istituto Ortopedico Rizzoli, Bologna, Italy

EUGENIO CAMMISA, MD
II Clinica Ortopedica e Traumatologica, Istituto Ortopedico Rizzoli, Bologna, Italy

CHRISTOPHER L. CAMP, MD
Department of Orthopedic Surgery and Sports Medicine, Mayo Clinic, Rochester, Minnesota, USA

ANTONINO CANTIVALLI, MD
University of Torino, Torino, Italy

BRIAN J. COLE, MD, MBA
Associate Chairman and Professor, Department of Orthopedic Surgery, Rush University Medical Center, Chairman, Department of Surgery, Rush Oak Park Hospital, Chicago, Illinois, USA

UMBERTO COTTINO, MD
Department of Orthopaedics and Traumatology, AO Ordine Mauriziano Hospital, University of Torino, Torino, Italy

MOLLY DAY, MD, ATC
Orthopedic Surgery Resident, PGY-4, Department of Orthopedics and Rehabilitation, University of Iowa Hospitals and Clinics, Iowa City, Iowa, USA

NICHOLAS C. DUETHMAN, MD
Department of Orthopedic Surgery and Sports Medicine, Mayo Clinic, Rochester, Minnesota, USA

STEFANO FRATINI, MD
II Clinica Ortopedica e Traumatologica, Istituto Ortopedico Rizzoli, Bologna, Italy

ALAN GETGOOD, MPhil, MD, FRCS(Tr&Orth)
Fowler Kennedy Sport Medicine Clinic, Western University, London, Ontario, Canada

J. ROBERT GIFFIN, MD, FRCSC, MBA
Wolf Orthopaedic Biomechanics Laboratory, Fowler Kennedy Sport Medicine Clinic, Bone and Joint Institute, London Health Sciences Centre, University Hospital, School of Physical Therapy, Faculty of Health Sciences, Department of Surgery, Schulich School of Medicine and Dentistry, St. Joseph's Health Care London, Professor, Orthopaedic Surgery, Western University, London, Ontario, Canada

ANDREAS H. GOMOLL, MD
Division of Sports Medicine, Department of Orthopedic Surgery, Hospital for Special Surgery, New York, New York, USA

ALBERTO GRASSI, MD
II Clinica Ortopedica e Traumatologica, Istituto Ortopedico Rizzoli, Bologna, Italy

AARON J. KRYCH, MD
Department of Orthopedic Surgery and Sports Medicine, Mayo Clinic, Rochester, Minnesota, USA

KRISTYN M. LEITCH, PhD
Wolf Orthopaedic Biomechanics Laboratory, Fowler Kennedy Sport Medicine Clinic, Bone and Joint Institute, Western University, London Health Sciences Centre, University Hospital, London, Ontario, Canada

NATALIE L. LEONG, MD
Assistant Professor, Department of Orthopaedic Surgery, University of Maryland, Baltimore, Staff Physician, Veterans Affairs Maryland Healthcare System, Baltimore, Maryland, USA

JOSEPH N. LIU, MD
Department of Orthopedic Surgery, Loma Linda Medical Center, Loma Linda, California, USA

AMANDA L. LORBERGS, PhD
Wolf Orthopaedic Biomechanics Laboratory, Fowler Kennedy Sport Medicine Clinic, Bone and Joint Institute, Western University, London Health Sciences Centre, University Hospital, London, Ontario, Canada

GIULIO MARIA MARCHEGGIANI MUCCIOLI, MD, PhD
II Clinica Ortopedica e Traumatologica, Istituto Ortopedico Rizzoli, Lab Biomeccanica, Bologna, Italy

KENDAL A. MARRIOTT, PT, PhD
Wolf Orthopaedic Biomechanics Laboratory, Fowler Kennedy Sport Medicine Clinic, Bone and Joint Institute, Western University, London Health Sciences Centre, University Hospital, London, Ontario, Canada

DARLI MYAT, PhD
Sydney Orthopaedic Research Institute (SORI), Chatswood, New South Wales, Australia

THOMAS NERI, MD, PhD
Sydney Orthopaedic Research Institute (SORI), Chatswood, New South Wales, Australia

ROCCO PAPALIA, MD, PhD
Department of Orthopedic and Trauma Surgery, University Campus Bio-Medico of Rome, Rome, Italy

DAVID PARKER, BMedSci, MBBS, FRACS, FAOrthA
Sydney Orthopaedic Research Institute (SORI), Chatswood, New South Wales, Australia

CAROLA PILONE, MD
Department of Orthopaedics and Traumatology, AO Ordine Mauriziano Hospital, University of Torino, Torino, Italy

CODIE A. PRIMEAU, MSc
Wolf Orthopaedic Biomechanics Laboratory, Fowler Kennedy Sport Medicine Clinic, Bone and Joint Institute, London Health Sciences Centre, University Hospital, School of Physical Therapy, Faculty of Health Sciences, Western University, London, Ontario, Canada

PHILIP P. ROESSLER, MD
Fowler Kennedy Sport Medicine Clinic, Western University, London, Ontario, Canada

ROBERTO ROSSI, MD
Department of Orthopaedics and Traumatology, AO Ordine Mauriziano Hospital, University of Torino, Torino, Italy

FEDERICA ROSSO, MD
Department of Orthopaedics and Traumatology, AO Ordine Mauriziano Hospital, University of Torino, Torino, Italy

TAYLOR M. SOUTHWORTH, BS
Research Assistant, Department of Orthopedic Surgery, Rush University Medical Center, Chicago, Illinois, USA

MICHAEL J. STUART, MD
Department of Orthopedic Surgery and Sports Medicine, Mayo Clinic, Rochester, Minnesota, USA

VITTORIO VACCARI, MD
II Clinica Ortopedica e Traumatologica, Istituto Ortopedico Rizzoli, Bologna, Italy

SEBASTIANO VASTA, MD
Department of Orthopedic and Trauma Surgery, University Campus Bio-Medico of Rome, Rome, Italy

BRIAN R. WOLF, MD, MS
John and Kim Callaghan Endowed Chair, Director of UI Sports Medicine, Professor, Vice-Chairman of Finance and Academic Affairs, Department of Orthopedics and Rehabilitation, University of Iowa Hospitals and Clinics, Head Team Physician, University of Iowa Athletics, Iowa City, Iowa, USA

STEFANO ZAFFAGNINI, MD
II Clinica Ortopedica e Traumatologica, Istituto Ortopedico Rizzoli, Bologna, Italy

BIAGIO ZAMPOGNA, MD
Department of Orthopedic and Trauma Surgery, University Campus Bio-Medico of Rome, Rome, Italy

Contents

Osteotomy is recognized as a knee joint–preserving surgical procedure to treat frontal and/or sagittal plane malalignment with or without associated instability. This article outlines the preoperative clinical and imaging assessments of prospective patients undergoing osteotomy. In addition, indications and contraindications as well as surgical planning are presented.

Observational studies suggest high tibial osteotomy produces substantial improvements in knee loading and stability that can limit the progression of joint damage; decrease pain; improve function and quality of life; and delay the need for knee replacement surgery. It can be cost-effective in knee osteoarthritis. However, systematic reviews and clinical practice guidelines are unable to provide strong recommendations, because limited high-level evidence supports its therapeutic value versus other treatments. We describe findings suggesting it can improve outcomes important to knee joint structure and function, patient quality of life, and health care systems. Future clinical trials are warranted and required.

Medial opening-wedge high tibial osteotomy has become increasingly popular for treating isolated, medial compartment arthrosis in younger, more active patients. Relative indications include age younger than 55 to 60 years, normal weight, preserved range of motion, and isolated medial compartment osteoarthritis or overload. Several surgical techniques exist for stabilization of the osteotomy with similar outcomes. Complication rates after medial opening-wedge high tibial osteotomy vary from 29% to 37%, with highest risk of nonunion, fracture, stiffness, and loss of correction. Good long-term outcomes can be achieved, with 5- and 10-year survivorship rates ranging from 75% to 98.7% and 51% to 97.6%, respectively.

Degenerative medial meniscal tears (DMMTs) are a common feature of early knee osteoarthritis (OA). Varus alignment is a strong risk factor for medial compartment knee OA and its progression. We propose that high tibial osteotomy (HTO) should be considered much earlier in the treatment algorithm for patients presenting with recurring medial knee pain, varus alignment, and DMMT, absent of radiographic OA. We provide rationale for investigating HTO as a disease-modifying intervention for secondary prevention in knee OA, and present case examples as low-level proof of principle. Finally, caveats and challenges are discussed along with proposed future research.

CLINICS IN SPORTS MEDICINE

THE CLINICS ARE AVAILABLE ONLINE!
Access your subscription at:
www.theclinics.com

CLINICS IN SPORTS MEDICINE

SERIES OF RELATED INTEREST

Orthopedic Clinics
Foot and Ankle Clinics
Hand Clinics
Physical Medicine and Rehabilitation Clinics
Clinics in Podiatric Medicine and Surgery

Foreword

Knee Osteotomies: A Powerful Tool

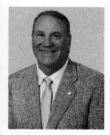

Mark D. Miller, MD
Consulting Editor

A wedge is one of six classical simple machines originally described by Archimedes and further refined during the Renaissance era. Simple machines provide a mechanical advantage, and the wedge has been characterized as the most powerful of these simple machines or tools. According to *Wikipedia*, a wedge "…can be used to separate two objects or portions of an object, lift up an object, or hold an object in place". Osteotomies are based on this simple tool, and, when used thoughtfully and carefully, can have powerful results. However, like any tool, a wedge used improperly can have deleterious effects.

I can think of no two individuals that are more knowledgeable about this subject than Drs Ned Amendola and Davide Bonasia. Dr Amendola has been teaching me (and, for that matter, many of us) about osteotomies for decades. Dr Amendola, now Chief of Sports Medicine at our rival ACC school Duke, trained and taught in London, Ontario, Canada, which is what I would consider "The Osteotomy University" of North America. His co-editor, Dr Bonasia, is an internationally recognized expert on knee osteotomies from AO Ordine Mauriziano "Umberto I" Hospital, University of Torino, Italy. I am pleased that together they have taken this issue of *Clinics in Sports Medicine* to a new level.

This issue covers the gamut of osteotomies of the knee. Opening, closing, medial, lateral, tibial, femoral…you name it, and it is here, and all from experts in the field.

Clin Sports Med 38 (2019) xiii–xiv
https://doi.org/10.1016/j.csm.2019.03.002
0278-5919/19/© 2019 Published by Elsevier Inc.

sportsmed.theclinics.com

So, I encourage you to read and study this issue of *Clinics in Sports Medicine* and apply this simple machine to complex problems about the knee in your practice.

Mark D. Miller, MD
Division of Sports Medicine
Department of Orthopaedic Surgery
University of Virginia
James Madison University
400 Ray C. Hunt Drive, Suite 330
Charlottesville, VA 22908-0159, USA

E-mail address:
mdm3p@virginia.edu

Preface

Limb Alignment: The Key to Success

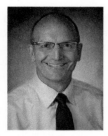 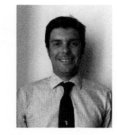

Annunziato (Ned) Amendola, MD   Davide Edoardo Bonasia, MD
Editors

In the young active patient with early knee osteoarthritis, chondral defects, meniscal deficiency, and/or ligament instability, it is crucial to assess knee alignment. In this issue of *Clinics in Sports Medicine*, you will appreciate the importance of limb alignment and how it is central to biologic reconstruction around the knee. It is important to have an armamentarium of techniques for the varus and valgus knees, meniscal transplantation combined with osteotomy, anterior cruciate ligament instability, and osteotomy. Each article is designed to be concise, give all the pertinent details, and really give the reader an opportunity to learn all aspects of the procedure. Although osteotomies have been around for a long time, the indications and techniques have improved, yielding more predictable results. In addition to the standard techniques currently utilized, we have included an article on navigation (Parker and colleagues) and accuracy of limb realignment. In many situations, especially with osteoarthritis, the disease process is already quite advanced. We all realize the outcome of osteotomy is dependent on the condition of the knee joint and yields poorer results in advanced osteoarthritis. Therefore, consideration and assessment for joint overload and earlier diagnosis and indications before advanced changes may be the way we should be looking at things, as in the article by Giffin and colleagues, "Degenerative meniscal tears and high tibial osteotomy." Do current treatment algorithms need to be realigned?" This special issue of *Clinics in Sports Medicine* has assembled experts from around the world to draw an overview of the use of osteotomy, patient evaluation,

Clin Sports Med 38 (2019) xv–xvi
https://doi.org/10.1016/j.csm.2019.03.001
0278-5919/19/© 2019 Published by Elsevier Inc.

techniques, indications, and results, aiming to provide up-to-date information on a hot topic that seems to be always in continuous development.

Annunziato (Ned) Amendola, MD
Urbaniak Sports Sciences Institute
Duke University
3475 Erwin Road
Durham, NC 27705, USA

Davide Edoardo Bonasia, MD
Department of Orthopaedics and Traumatology
AO Ordine Mauriziano "Umberto I" Hospital
University of Torino
Via LAmarmora 26
10128, Torino, Italy

E-mail addresses:
ned.amendola@duke.edu (A. Amendola)
davidebonasia@virgilio.it (D.E. Bonasia)

Patient Evaluation and Indications for Osteotomy Around the Knee

Biagio Zampogna, MD, Sebastiano Vasta, MD*,
Rocco Papalia, MD, PhD

KEYWORDS

- Unicompartmental knee osteoarthritis • Joint preservation • Knee osteotomy
- High tibial osteotomy (HTO) • Distal femoral osteotomy (DFO) • Osteotomy planning
- Radiographs

KEY POINTS

- Osteotomies around the knee are an excellent surgical joint-preservation option in treating frontal and/or sagittal plane malalignment with or without associated instability.
- Success depends on accurate preoperative patient assessment, through history taking and physical examination and meticulous preoperative planning on a complete radiologic series.
- Extra-articular deformity has been considered as a sine qua non criterion for osteotomies.
- Intra-articular malalignment, secondary to full cartilage loss and/or partial or total meniscectomy, is best addressed by unicompartmental knee replacement.
- Performing osteotomy with the appropriate indications and adhesions to ideal criteria helps in reaching satisfactory outcomes.

INTRODUCTION

Osteotomy is recognized as a knee joint–preserving surgical procedure to treat frontal and/or sagittal plane malalignment with or without associated instability. The principal aims of such procedures are correction of the frontal and/or sagittal plane malalignment, protection of cartilage, and optimization of coronal and anteroposterior knee stability.[1] High tibial osteotomy (HTO) is considered a viable solution for symptomatic varus knee caused by constitutional or post-traumatic metaphyseal deformity.[2] Valgus knee with mechanical overload on lateral compartment can be managed by distal femoral osteotomy (DFO).[3] Knee instability, produced by sagittal bony

Disclosure: The authors do not have anything to disclose with regard to the article content.
Department of Orthopedic and Trauma Surgery, University Campus Bio-Medico of Rome, Via Alvaro del Portillo, 200, Rome 00128, Italy
* Corresponding author.
E-mail address: sebastianovasta@hotmail.it

imbalance, represents a peculiar and not well-known disorder that may be addressed by pure sagittal or frontal combined osteotomies.[4] A correct preoperative evaluation requires meticulous clinical examination combined with a complete radiologic examination series including traditional radiographs and MRI.[2] This article outlines the preoperative clinical and imaging assessments of these cases. In addition, indications and contraindications as well as surgical planning are presented.

CLINICAL EVALUATION

An accurate history of the patient has to be taken to assess the following information[2,5,6]:

1. Age and occupation
2. Level of activity
3. Medical history with general health comorbidity
4. History of previous surgery of the affected knee
5. Symptoms history (type and timing of pain, locking or instability episodes)
6. Previous conservative treatment of the affected knee
7. Patient expectations on postoperative activity level

Physical examination should start with a stand-up and gait 3 planar assessment of general lower limb alignment, occurrence of thrust on the affected side, and presence of rotational deformity. Subsequently a bench clinical examination is necessary to focus on[2,5,6]:

1. Starter knee examination (limb discrepancy, presence of effusion or crepitus)
2. Range of motion (ROM) measurement (possible flexion contracture)
3. Deformity (fixed or correctable) and knee stability (frontal, sagittal, and rotational plane) assessment
4. Tenderness at joint line (possible meniscal tears), tibial plateau, and femoral condyle
5. Patellar tracking evaluation and facet tenderness
6. Homolateral hip and ankle examination
7. Presence of neurovascular alterations

RADIOLOGIC EVALUATION

Radiologic assessment maintains a key role both in indications and surgical planning. An accurate radiologic evaluation relies on a complete series of radiographs[2,5,6]:

1. Bilateral full-length weight-bearing view (bipodalic stance and monopodalic stance for the limb of interest)
2. Anteroposterior and lateral weight-bearing views
3. Posteroanterior views at 45° of flexion (Rosenberg views)
4. Skyline views

Preoperative surgical planning is performed on bilateral full-length weight-bearing plain radiograph view.[7] Lateral views are necessary for tibial slope[8] and patellar height calculation (Insall-Salvati, Blackburne-Peel, or Caton-Deschamps index).[9] Every realignment surgery requires an MRI evaluation to check the status of the following structures:

1. Cartilage and subchondral bone
2. Ligaments and tendons
3. Menisci

INDICATIONS AND CONTRAINDICATIONS

The aim of an osteotomy is to correct a bone deformity redistribute loads across the joint. Coronal malalignment results in medial or lateral compartment overload, leading to cartilage wear, which will decrease the medial or lateral joint space, further increasing malalignment and therefore compartment overload. Osteotomies are thus a good option to break this vicious circle.[10] However, unicompartmental overload secondary to coronal malalignment is not the only indication to osteotomy. Osteotomies have gained interest also to modify the sagittal plane, by acting on tibial slope, in the setting of ligament imbalance: chronic anterior cruciate ligament injury (ACL) associated with varus malalignment,[11] chronic posterolateral corner (PLC), and posterior cruciate ligament (PCL) ± ACL associated with varus malalignment (a condition known also as double varus, or triple varus if there is concomitant recurvatum).[12] The sagittal plane should also be considered. In fact, sagittal imbalance could be secondary to bony deformity or ligament deficiency. Increased tibial slope has been correlated with increased strain on the ACL, putting the native ligament or the graft at higher risk of rupture.[13] Cartilage procedures (such as autograft or allograft transplantation) or meniscal allograft transplantation (MAT) in the setting of a coronal malalignment could result in poor outcomes. Combining knee realignment with a biological procedure or MAT may help to improve patient outcomes.[14]

General indications for osteotomies around the knee[10]

1. Malalignment and arthritis

2. Malalignment and instability

3. Malalignment with arthritis and instability

4. Malalignment with chondral or meniscal allografts

Data from McNamara I, Birmingham TB, Fowler PJ, et al. High tibial osteotomy: evolution of research and clinical applications—a Canadian experience. Knee Surg Sports Traumatol Arthrosc 2013;21:23–31.

Ideal Criteria for Knee Osteotomies on the Coronal Plane

When considering osteotomies around the knee, the following are ideal criteria:

Clinical conditions

1. Pain located at one single tibiofemoral compartment
2. Nonreducible deformity (coronal deformity that is not only due to intra-articular deformity)
3. Full to good ROM (5°–10° of flexion contracture can be tolerated in selected cases)

Radiologic conditions

1. Joint space narrowing (partial or total) of one compartment
2. Extra-articular deformity (>5°)

Contraindications

1. Involvement of multiple compartments
2. Inflammatory arthritis
3. Absence of bony deformity

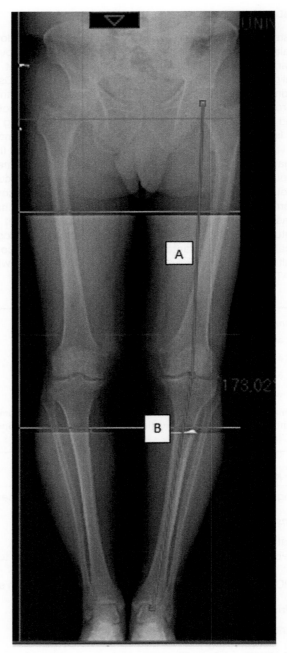

Fig. 1. Long leg view, bipodalic stance. (*A*) Femur mechanical axis. (*B*) Tibial mechanical axis. The hip-knee-ankle (HKA) angle is about 7°, in varus.

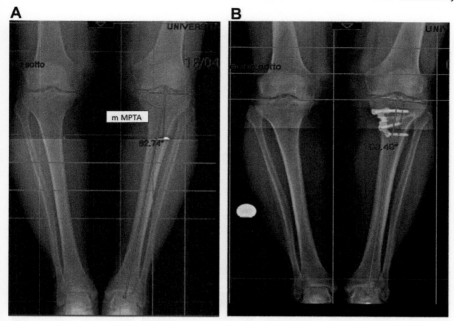

Fig. 2. Long leg view, focused on the tibia. (*A*) preoperative mechanical medial proximal tibial angle (mMPTA). (*B*) Postoperative view after HTO. Notice how the mMPTA improved to 90°.

Extra-articular deformity has been considered as a sine qua non criterion for osteotomies. In fact, Lobenhoffer[1] strongly recommends that at least one of the joint angles (lateral distal femoral angle, medial proximal tibial angle) is altered. When malalignment is intra-articular, secondary to full cartilage loss and/or partial or total meniscectomy, joint angles are within normal ranges, despite an overall malalignment. This condition is best addressed by unicompartmental knee replacement (UKA).[1] Age, obesity, and asymptomatic/mild symptomatic patellar-femoral changes are relative contraindications.[1] Outcomes from studies in Asian countries have shown that age and severe osteoarthritis with Kellgren-Lawrence (KL) grade IV are no longer contraindications to osteotomy.[15,16] In addition, a retrospective study of 533 patients demonstrated favorable outcomes of opening wedge high tibial osteotomy (HTO) even in obese patients.[17] Regarding sagittal plane deformity, current literature suggests performing an anterior closing wedge osteotomy of the proximal tibia (tibial deflexion osteotomy) in the case of ACL (second) revision surgery and greater than 12° posterior tibial slope.[4] An anterior opening wedge osteotomy of the proximal tibia (antirecurvatum, tibial flexion osteotomy) is indicated when there is a symptomatic (pain, instability) genu recurvatum with inverted posterior tibial slope and/or ligament deficiencies. If recurvatum is secondary to capsuloligamentous traumatic insufficiency without bony deformity, there is less rationale for a tibial flexion osteotomy, although it could protect the reconstructed ligaments.[18]

Indications for sagittal plane osteotomy[18]:

Tibial deflexion osteotomy

1. Second or third ACL graft injury and posterior tibial slope greater than 12°

Tibial flexion osteotomy (antirecurvatum osteotomy)

2. PLC/PCL insufficiency and inverted tibial slope

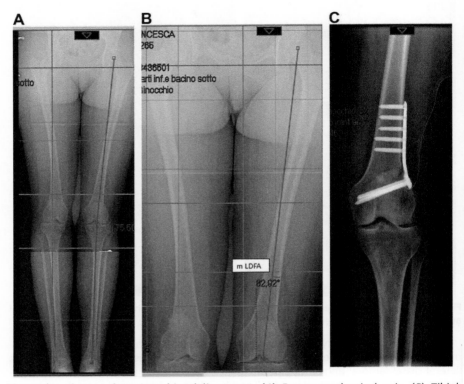

Fig. 3. (*A*, *B*) Long leg view, bipodalic stance. (*A*) Femur mechanical axis. (*B*) Tibial mechanical axis. The HKA angle is about 5° in valgus. Preoperative mechanical lateral distal femoral angle is significantly reduced. (*C*) Postoperative improved alignment after DFO.

Overall, when considering an osteotomy one nonclinical, nonradiologic, but an essential criterion is patient compliance. Osteotomy is a complex surgery, which requires a variable time of non–weight bearing or protected weight bearing, followed by an intense rehabilitation, to fully recover function. There is a risk for nonunion (up to 4.4%[19]) and for subsequent surgery such as knee replacement (5%–45%[20]). Possible risks and complications, as well as the postoperative indications, should be thoroughly discussed with the patient.

PREOPERATIVE WORKUP AND PLANNING

An accurate preoperative plan is necessary to reduce the risk for complications and failure of osteotomies. Excessive overcorrection can lead to unsatisfactory outcomes, whereas undercorrection can result in persisting symptoms. It is paramount to assess the status of the contralateral tibiofemoral compartment as well as the patellar-femoral one by MRI and/or arthroscopy before performing the osteotomy.[2] Lateral views are necessary to assess patella height. If severe patella baja is diagnosed, consider performing a tibial tubercle osteotomy in combination with opening wedge HTO, or consider a closing wedge osteotomy.[10] Lateral views are also necessary to measure posterior tibial slope. The optimal amount of

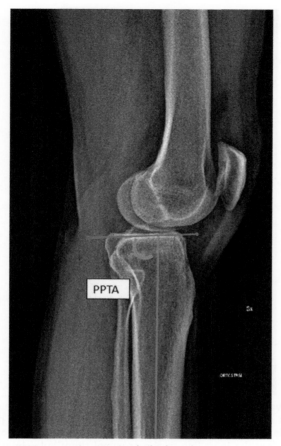

Fig. 4. Lateral view. PPTA, posterior proximal tibial angle.

correction should be accurately planned preoperatively. Several investigators[7,21,22] recommend a valgus-producing HTO, aiming to a point about 62.5% of tibial plateau, resulting in a mechanical axis with between 3° and 5° of valgus. This slight overcorrection is strongly recommended in cases of osteotomy for medial compartment arthritis.[23] Moreover, evidence that the weight-bearing line shifts progressively medially until 1 year postoperatively must be considered.[24] However, severe overcorrection can lead to poor outcomes in terms of unsatisfactory cosmetics and lateral compartment overload.[25] Therefore, some investigators have proposed a personalized approach depending on the pathology that must be addressed. In cases of more severe grades of osteoarthritis (KL grade III and IV), surgeons should aim for a point at 60% to 65%. A milder degree of osteoarthritis or osteotomies associated with MAT could aim for a point at 50% to 60%.[26] Regarding distal femur osteotomy to correct a valgus alignment, surgeons should aim for an osteotomy producing a neutral mechanical axis. Overcorrection in varus-producing osteotomies is contraindicated.[3] Over time several methods for preoperative planning have been developed, based on either the anatomic or mechanical axes.[25,27–31]

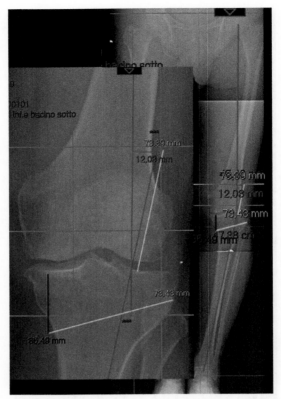

Fig. 5. Preoperative planning for a valgus-producing opening wedge high tibial osteotomy. Green lines correspond to femur and tibial mechanical axes passing through 62.5% of the tibia width. Yellow line on the tibia indicates the osteotomy line, from a point 3.5 cm below the joint line to the proximal tibiofibular joint. This line is reported on the tibial mechanical axes, starting from the apex of the HKA. The resulting distance as measured by the red line corresponds to the opening that should be achieved.

Essential joint angles that should be calculated are as follows (**Figs. 1–4**)[32]:

1. mMPTA: mechanical medial proximal tibial angle (normal 87°, range 85°–90°)
2. mLDFA: mechanical lateral distal femoral angle (normal 88°, range 85°–90°)
3. PPTA: posterior proximal tibial angle (normal 81°, range 77°–84°)

The authors commonly use the method described by Dugdale and colleagues[7] (**Figs. 5** and **6** explain the methods). The overall limb alignment should be assessed, drawing a line from the center of the femoral head to the center of the knee (femur mechanical axis) and from the center of the knee to the center of the tibiotalar joint (tibial mechanical axis) (**Figs. 5** and **6**).

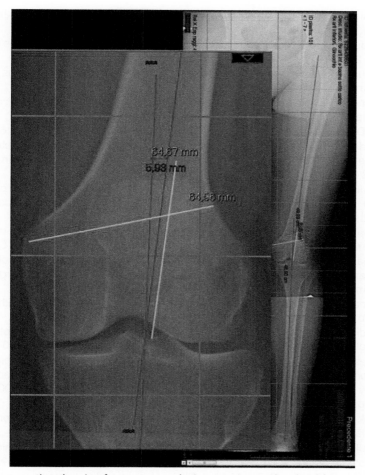

Fig. 6. Preoperative planning for a varus-producing opening wedge distal femur osteotomy. Green lines correspond to femur and tibial mechanical axes passing through the center of the knee. Yellow line indicates osteotomy line, which is reported on the tibial mechanical axes, starting from the apex of the HKA. The resulting distance as measured by the red line corresponds to the opening that should be achieved.

SUMMARY

Osteotomies around the knee represent an excellent surgical joint-preservation option. Success depends on accurate preoperative patient assessment, thorough history taking and physical examination, and meticulous preoperative planning on a complete radiographic series. Performing osteotomy with the appropriate indications and adherence to ideal criteria helps in reaching satisfactory outcomes.

REFERENCES

1. Lobenhoffer P. Indication for unicompartmental knee replacement versus osteotomy around the knee. J Knee Surg 2017;30:769–73.

2. Rossi R, Bonasia DE, Amendola A. The role of high tibial osteotomy in the varus knee. J Am Acad Orthop Surg 2011;19:590–9.
3. Puddu G, Cipolla M, Cerullo G, et al. Which osteotomy for a valgus knee? Int Orthop 2010;34:239–47.
4. Dejour D, La Barbera G, Pasqualotto S, et al. Sagittal plane corrections around the knee. J Knee Surg 2017;30:736–45.
5. Amendola A, Panarella L. High tibial osteotomy for the treatment of unicompartmental arthritis of the knee. Orthop Clin North Am 2005;36:497–504.
6. Lee DC, Byun SJ. High tibial osteotomy. Knee Surg Relat Res 2012;24:61–9.
7. Dugdale TW, Noyes FR, Styer D. Preoperative planning for high tibial osteotomy. The effect of lateral tibiofemoral separation and tibiofemoral length. Clin Orthop 1992;(274):248–64.
8. Yoo JH, Chang CB, Shin KS, et al. Anatomical references to assess the posterior tibial slope in total knee arthroplasty: a comparison of 5 anatomical axes. J Arthroplasty 2008;23:586–92.
9. Phillips CL, Silver D a T, Schranz PJ, et al. The measurement of patellar height: a review of the methods of imaging. J Bone Joint Surg Br 2010;92:1045–53.
10. McNamara I, Birmingham TB, Fowler PJ, et al. High tibial osteotomy: evolution of research and clinical applications—a Canadian experience. Knee Surg Sports Traumatol Arthrosc 2013;21:23–31.
11. Herman BV, Giffin JR. High tibial osteotomy in the ACL-deficient knee with medial compartment osteoarthritis. J Orthop Traumatol 2016;17:277–85.
12. Naudie DDR, Amendola A, Fowler PJ. Opening wedge high tibial osteotomy for symptomatic hyperextension-varus thrust. Am J Sports Med 2004;32:60–70.
13. Agneskirchner JD, Hurschler C, Stukenborg-Colsman C, et al. Effect of high tibial flexion osteotomy on cartilage pressure and joint kinematics: a biomechanical study in human cadaveric knees. Winner of the AGA-DonJoy Award 2004. Arch Orthop Trauma Surg 2004;124:575–84.
14. Frank RM, Cotter EJ, Strauss EJ, et al. The utility of biologics, osteotomy, and cartilage restoration in the knee. J Am Acad Orthop Surg 2018;26:e11–25.
15. Akizuki S, Shibakawa A, Takizawa T, et al. The long-term outcome of high tibial osteotomy: a ten- to 20-year follow-up. J Bone Joint Surg Br 2008;90:592–6.
16. Takeuchi R, Aratake M, Bito H, et al. Clinical results and radiographical evaluation of opening wedge high tibial osteotomy for spontaneous osteonecrosis of the knee. Knee Surg Sports Traumatol Arthrosc 2009;17:361–8.
17. Floerkemeier S, Staubli AE, Schroeter S, et al. Does obesity and nicotine abuse influence the outcome and complication rate after open-wedge high tibial osteotomy? A retrospective evaluation of five hundred and thirty three patients. Int Orthop 2014;38:55–60.
18. Dejour D, Bonin N, Locatelli E. Tibial antirecurvatum osteotomies. Oper Tech Sports Med 2000;8:67–70.
19. Spahn G. Complications in high tibial (medial opening wedge) osteotomy. Arch Orthop Trauma Surg 2004;124:649–53.
20. Amendola A, Bonasia DE. Results of high tibial osteotomy: review of the literature. Int Orthop 2010;34:155–60.
21. Miniaci A, Ballmer FT, Ballmer PM, et al. Proximal tibial osteotomy. A new fixation device. Clin Orthop Relat Res 1989;(246):250–9.
22. Noyes FR, Barber SD, Simon R. High tibial osteotomy and ligament reconstruction in varus angulated, anterior cruciate ligament-deficient knees. A two- to seven-year follow-up study. Am J Sports Med 1993;21:2–12.

23. Kumagai K, Akamatsu Y, Kobayashi H, et al. Factors affecting cartilage repair after medial opening-wedge high tibial osteotomy. Knee Surg Sports Traumatol Arthrosc 2017;25:779–84.
24. Lee YS, Lee BK, Kwon JH, et al. Serial assessment of weight-bearing lower extremity alignment radiographs after open-wedge high tibial osteotomy. Arthroscopy 2014;30:319–25.
25. Hernigou P, Medevielle D, Debeyre J, et al. Proximal tibial osteotomy for osteoarthritis with varus deformity. A ten to thirteen-year follow-up study. J Bone Joint Surg Am 1987;69:332–54.
26. Feucht MJ, Minzlaff P, Saier T, et al. Degree of axis correction in valgus high tibial osteotomy: proposal of an individualised approach. Int Orthop 2014;38:2273–80.
27. Engel GM, Lippert FG. Valgus tibial osteotomy: avoiding the pitfalls. Clin Orthop Relat Res 1981;(160):137–43.
28. Kettelkamp DB, Wenger DR, Chao EY, et al. Results of proximal tibial osteotomy. The effects of tibiofemoral angle, stance-phase flexion-extension, and medial-plateau force. J Bone Joint Surg Am 1976;58:952–60.
29. Coventry MB. Upper tibial osteotomy for osteoarthritis. J Bone Joint Surg Am 1985;67:1136–40.
30. Koshino T, Morii T, Wada J, et al. High tibial osteotomy with fixation by a blade plate for medial compartment osteoarthritis of the knee. Orthop Clin North Am 1989;20:227–43.
31. Myrnerts R. Optimal correction in high tibial osteotomy for varus deformity. Acta Orthop Scand 1980;51:689–94.
32. Paley D. Principles of deformity correction. Berlin and Heidelberg: Springer-Verlag; 2002.

Improved Methods to Measure Outcomes After High Tibial Osteotomy

Amanda L. Lorbergs, PhD[a,b], Trevor B. Birmingham, PT, PhD[a,b,c],*,
Codie A. Primeau, MSc[a,b,c], Hayden F. Atkinson, BSc[a,b,c],
Kendal A. Marriott, PT, PhD[a,b],
J. Robert Giffin, MD, FRCSC, MBA[a,b,c,d],*

KEYWORDS

- High tibial osteotomy • Outcome measures • Evidence-based practice
- Knee osteoarthritis • Varus gonarthrosis

KEY POINTS

- Second-look arthroscopy and quantitative MRI show regeneration of articular cartilage is possible after high tibial osteotomy.
- Large mean improvements in the distribution of knee load during walking are observed 10 years after high tibial osteotomy.
- Meta-analysis also suggests large mean improvements in patient-reported outcomes that extend beyond 10 years after surgery.
- Despite these findings from observational studies, high tibial osteotomy is seldom recommended in evidence-based guidelines and rates of high tibial osteotomy are comparatively low and decreasing.
- Higher level evidence comparing high tibial osteotomy with alternate treatments using the best available methods is both warranted and required for high tibial osteotomy to have a greater impact.

Disclosures: The authors have no disclosures to declare related to this work.
[a] Wolf Orthopaedic Biomechanics Laboratory, Fowler Kennedy Sport Medicine Clinic, University of Western Ontario, 3M Centre, Room 1220, London, Ontario N6A 3K7, Canada; [b] Bone and Joint Institute, University of Western Ontario, London Health Sciences Centre, University Hospital B6-200, London, Ontario N6A 5B5, Canada; [c] School of Physical Therapy, Faculty of Health Sciences, University of Western Ontario, 1201 Western Rd, London, Ontario N6G 1H1, Canada; [d] Department of Surgery, Schulich School of Medicine and Dentistry, University of Ontario, St. Joseph's Healthcare London, 268 Grosvenor St, London, Ontario N6A 4V2, Canada
* Corresponding authors. Wolf Orthopaedic Biomechanics Laboratory, Fowler Kennedy Sport Medicine Clinic, University of Western Ontario, 3M Centre, Room 1220, London, Ontario N6A 3K7, Canada.
E-mail addresses: tbirming@uwo.ca (T.B.B.); rgiffin@uwo.ca (J.R.G.)

Clin Sports Med 38 (2019) 317–329
https://doi.org/10.1016/j.csm.2019.02.001
sportsmed.theclinics.com

INTRODUCTION

Limb realignment surgery, particularly high tibial osteotomy (HTO), is most often described as a treatment option for relatively young, active patients with well-established knee osteoarthritis (OA) isolated to one compartment, and for whom total joint replacement is unwarranted.[1] Other investigators suggest that the indications for HTO are considerably broader and the surgery can produce favorable results for patients with a greater range of disease characteristics, severities, and ages.[2] Moreover, limb realignment surgery is increasingly being considered for patients with knee instability[3] and as a concomitant treatment to other joint preservation therapies.[4] Accordingly, limb realignment procedures should be appropriate for a large segment of the population who have knee pathology, yet rates are much lower and decreasing compared with other knee surgeries.[5–7] Despite several observational studies, systematic reviews[8] and clinical practice guidelines[9] are unable to provide strong recommendations for HTO because there is limited high-level evidence to support the therapeutic value of the procedures. The purpose of this article is to describe the results from selected observational studies, ranging from case series to population-based studies, that suggest that limb realignment can substantially improve outcome measures important to knee joint structure and function, patient quality of life, and health care systems. Our intent is to highlight the potent positive effects that HTO can produce and encourage future clinical trials that use similar outcome measures to compare the procedure to other interventions.

LEVELS OF EVIDENCE

Orthopedic clinical practice guidelines rely on the well-accepted levels of evidence for therapeutic studies evaluating the results of treatment.[10] Randomized, clinical trials are considered high-level evidence, whereas observational studies without a comparison with a control or another treatment are considered low-level evidence. Several laboratory investigations, single-group prospective cohorts and population-based studies investigating HTO do indeed exist. These observational studies have advanced knowledge about surgical and rehabilitation techniques, potential prognostic factors, survivorship, rates of use, and cost-effectiveness models. However, very few randomized trials have compared HTO with alternative treatments. The randomized trials that do exist have relatively limited eligibility criteria because they typically compare other, relatively uncommon, surgical techniques with one another (eg, HTO vs unicompartmental arthroplasty, HTO vs knee joint distraction, or joint preservation therapies with or without HTO). Limb realignment surgery may provide the opportunity to improve outcomes in a much larger segment of the population with knee OA. Future randomized trials that compare limb realignment surgery with other, more commonly recommended treatments for similar patients are required to demonstrate the potential therapeutic value of the procedure. Planning such studies should benefit from the several types of outcome measures previously used in observational studies of HTO that suggest encouraging results for joint, patient, and economic outcomes.

OUTCOME MEASURES
Knee Loading

Several 3-dimensional gait studies demonstrate HTO produces long-term improvements in knee loading during walking, represented as changes in the external knee moments in all 3 planes of motion.[11–14] The knee adduction moment, a proxy for the mediolateral distribution of knee load, has been particularly well-studied, with very large mean reductions (approximately 50%) consistently reported 6 months and 1, 2, and 5 years after the initial procedure,[2,12,15,16] and with substantial reductions (approximately 40%) sustained as long as 10 years after surgery (**Fig. 1**). The size of these changes deserves emphasis as it is substantially higher than changes observed while using other devices intended to alter medial knee loading, such as an unloader brace or a lateral heel wedge.[17] There also seems to be less need for muscle co-contraction across the knee after HTO, although this factor may depend on whether the target correction is achieved.[18] Importantly, decreases in the knee adduction moment during walking seem to influence results after HTO,[2,19] although the association may not be straightforward. For example, recent data suggest that, when divided into quartiles, although all strata improved significantly, patients with neither the largest nor the smallest changes in adduction moment had the highest 5-year improvements in patient-reported outcomes.[2]

Limitations in relying largely on the changes in external knee moments must be acknowledged. More sophisticated methods to measure and/or model the actual loads on the knee compartments in vivo, including muscular contributions, coupled with more advanced imaging methods may provide a greater understanding of the types of biomechanical changes achievable with HTO. For example, although dynamic radiography (ie, single and biplane fluoroscopy) has been used to study the arthrokinematics associated with posterior cruciate ligament insufficiency and the effects of unloader knee bracing,[20,21] they have not been used to investigate HTO. These studies suggest fluoroscopy can detect very small changes in joint kinematics during ambulation (eg, walking, stair ascent). For example, measuring the condylar separation of the knee joint space during walking could be measured with an accuracy of 0.5 mm. Fluoroscopy-enabled evaluation of micromotion after HTO may provide an opportunity to better understand the more subtle biomechanical changes achieved. Regardless, given the association between the high knee adduction moment and medial tibiofemoral OA progression,[22] a large, sustained reduction after HTO supports the biomechanical rationale for limb realignment as a disease-modifying intervention, and provides incentive to investigate the link between changes in joint biomechanics and measures of joint damage and repair.

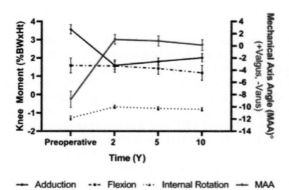

Fig. 1. Means with 95% confidence intervals for peak external knee moments during walking (*left axis; black lines*) and mechanical axis angle during standing (*right axis; red line*) before and after medial opening HTO (unpublished data for 37 patients provided by the authors). BW, body weight; Ht, height.

Muscular Strength

Muscle strength and muscle activation can contribute to knee degeneration and can become further impaired by disuse and recovery from surgical intervention. For example, compared with healthy, age-matched individuals, individuals with medial tibiofemoral knee OA have decreased knee flexor and extensor muscle strength,[23] which carries over into the recovery phase after HTO.[24] Several studies suggest that postoperative strength gradually increases in the first year after surgery, leading to a recovery of the preoperative strength levels within 12 to 18 months after HTO.[23,25–27] Although postoperative muscle strength declines are likely unavoidable, Kean and colleagues[24] (2011) showed that a 12-week preoperative exercise program focused on increasing hamstrings and quadriceps strength can help improve the Knee injury and Osteoarthritis Outcome Score (KOOS) sport and recreation and activities of daily living subscales at 6 months after surgery. Additionally, significant improvements in knee symptoms and function measured by the Lysholm score (knee-specific questionnaire) and the International Knee Documentation Committee Subjective Knee Evaluation were observed at 12 months after HTO, yet improvements in function continued between 12 and 24 months after HTO.[25] Predicting postsurgical pain and functional deficits is not well-understood; however, preoperative and postoperative muscle strengthening is paramount for preparing for surgery and regaining function after limb realignment. Thus, neuromuscular retraining and muscle strengthening is recommended as a part of HTO standard of care.

Articular Cartilage and Biomarkers

A limited number of studies have directly investigated the ability of HTO to alter cartilage damage and repair, using either second-look arthroscopy or MRI. Small cohort studies, using second look arthroscopy, have shown tissue regeneration in the medial tibiofemoral compartment for more than half of patients (55%–91%; n = 59–159) at 12 months after valgus-producing HTO.[28–30] Detecting longitudinal changes in the quantitative measures of articular cartilage are also possible. For example, MRI shows considerable promise in detecting very small decreases in knee articular cartilage thickness over as little as 6 months in patients with moderate knee OA.[31] Preliminary data, using cartilage segmentation and blinding outcome assessors to time point (**Fig. 2**) suggest that MRI can detect increases in the medial articular cartilage thickness after HTO that are associated with the redistribution of load away from the medial compartment.[32]

Other MRI techniques have also been used to assess the effect of HTO on articular cartilage, including measures of glycosaminoglycan content assessed via delayed gadolinium enhanced MRI of cartilage, and changes in bone metabolism via single-photon emission computed tomography and MRI. These studies suggest favorable changes after HTO, although the composition of regenerated seems appears to be more like fibrocartilage than hyaline cartilage.[33–35] Additionally, single-photon emission computed tomography and MRI data suggest improvements in other important measures in knee joint health after HTO, including decreased bone metabolism and a lower trabecular number in the medial tibiofemoral joint, indicative of a decreased load on the medial compartment and off-loaded subchondral bone.[36,37]

Candidate biochemical markers representative of cartilage degeneration and regeneration may also be quantified to describe potential articular cartilage responses after HTO.[38] Biomolecular advances suggest that inflammatory mediators also contribute to the cartilage degeneration process and may be altered after surgery.[39–41] The importance of assessing imaging and biochemical markers after limb realignment is

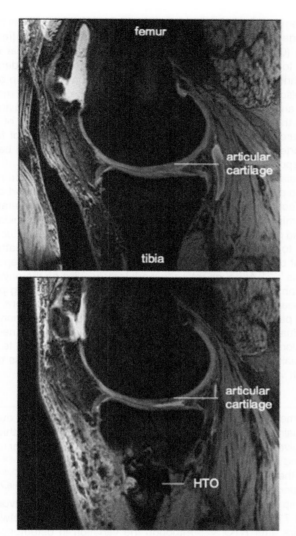

Fig. 2. Sagittal dual echo steady-state sequence[31,90] MRI scans of the medial tibiofemoral compartment before (top) and after (bottom) medial opening HTO using a polyether-ether-ketone plate. Minimal to no image artifact enables segmentation and quantification of articular cartilage thickness and morphology.

underscored by the fact the HTO is seldom considered by the larger arthritis community as a potential disease-modifying intervention. As the capabilities of advanced imaging techniques improve and become more readily available, they should be incorporated into comparative effectiveness studies evaluating HTO.

Patient-Reported Outcomes

The most common outcomes used to assess pain and physical function after HTO are the KOOS, the Short Form-12 Health Survey, and the Short Form-36 Health Survey.[2,8,42–49] These studies have shown large mean improvements by 12 months after

HTO, which seem to be sustained for at least 5 years.[1] For pain, the most common outcomes include the visual analogue scale (from 0 [no pain] to 10 [maximum pain]) and the KOOS (0–100 worst to best) pain domain. In studies that used a visual analogue scale to measure pain after HTO, activity-related pain is decreased in patients at 6, 12, and 24 months after surgery.[25] Longitudinal follow-up of HTO patient cohorts have also shown clinically meaningful decreases in pain, measured using the KOOS, at 2 and 5 years after HTO.[2,43] A meta-analysis by Spahn and colleagues[1] (2013) showed that HTO provided improvements using a variety of knee-specific outcome measures. Improvements from baseline to 5 to 8 years of follow-up after HTO were reported as a standardized mean difference of 5.0, and baseline to 9 to 12 years was reported as 1.7; both are very large effect sizes.

Important goals of treatment for patients undergoing HTO include pain relief, but prompt return to preoperative employment, daily activities, and sport or leisure have tremendous effects on quality of life. Regaining function of the operated limb is an important determinant of return to occupational activity. Although clinical research describes improved pain and function after HTO,[46,50,51] few published studies assess the patients' ability to return to preoperative work and sports activities after HTO.[52] The average amount of time off work after limb realignment surgery is reported between 13 and 23 weeks.[53–56] Although return to work largely relies on the physical demands of the occupation, osteotomy fixation also plays a role, with locking plates allowing earlier weight-bearing than nonlocking devices.[57–59] Common reasons for an inability to work include pain and poor range of motion.[55] In general, by 24 months after HTO, nearly all individuals report returning to work without limitations, yet knee symptoms in a small proportion of individuals may persist and discourage return to work.[55] Additionally, individuals with impaired mobility and psychological distress tend to require a longer time off work.[55,60]

Survivorship

A critical outcome of HTO is survivorship, most often defined as the duration that the osteotomy remains in situ without conversion to a total knee arthroplasty (TKA). Osteotomy survival is reported between 91% and 99% at 5 years after medial opening HTO[1,53,61–67] and between 73% and 94% for lateral closing HTO.[61,66,68] At 10 years postoperative, the survival range varies from 84% to 92%[1,5,7,61,65,68–72] for medial opening HTO, and from 51% to 85% for lateral closing HTO.[61,66,68,72] Most longer term survivorship reports are for lateral closing HTOs,[1] with survivorship reported from 39% and 71%[61,69] at 15 years, 51%[61] at 18 years, and between 30% and 50% at 20 years after HTO.[68,72] Although the variation in osteotomy type may or may not make a difference, it is important to note that lateral closing HTOs in these studies were performed on patients much later in their disease. As a result, the surgical intervention may not have been performed soon enough to be disease modifying and patients with medial opening HTOs are expected to have a prolonged effect of surgery and overall better survivorship compared with the cohort with lateral closing HTOs.

Adverse Events

Although patient satisfaction with HTO is relatively high,[73] the low rates of performing limb realignment for medial tibiofemoral knee OA may be partially due to reported complications associated with the procedure. Examples of common HTO complications include loss of correction (with or without hardware failure),[74,75] delayed union or nonunion,[76–78] and overcorrection,[25] with overall rates of complication ranging from 6% to 55%.[8,50,58,79–83] A meta-analysis by Spahn and colleagues[1] (2013) reported a complication event rate of 0.138 after HTO.

However, there are often disparities in how complications are reported in the literature. The severity of adverse events can be grouped based on how patients and health care professionals manage the complication, from relatively benign to severe. In a retrospective case series, Martin and colleagues[76] (2014) reviewed 323 HTOs performed on 292 patients (mean age, 46 years) using a nonlocking plate with complications grouped in 3 categories (class I, II, and III) based on severity and the treatment required. It may be beneficial to adopt a more universal way of reporting complications in a similar manner for transparency. The authors also identified that diabetic individuals and smokers (or ex-smokers) had double the rates of complication (ie, delayed union, nonunion) compared with those who were not, highlighting the importance of appropriate patient selection moving forward for decreasing the risk of complication.

Compared with lateral closing HTO, adverse event rates have been reported to be higher with medial opening HTO.[8,79,80] However, higher adverse event rates may have been reported as surgeons switched to an unfamiliar technique involving a learning curve and requiring a new understanding of adequate fixation options. Encouragingly, the more recent introduction of advanced plate technology is believed to have decreased adverse events with medial opening HTO. More rigorous study trial designs are warranted to investigate the impact these plate advancements have on the rate of complication after HTO.

Cost Effectiveness

The cost effectiveness of HTO compared with alternative interventions is another important consideration.[84,85] Economic evaluations compare both the costs and clinical effects of treatments simultaneously, providing an evaluative tool to make choices concerning the deployment of finances for maximum health benefit.[86]

Konopka and colleagues[85] (2015) evaluated the lifetime cost-effectiveness of HTO when compared with unicompartmental knee arthroplasty (UKA) and TKA in patients 50 to 60 years of age with medial tibiofemoral knee OA from a payer perspective (ie, procedure costs and health care resource use) using a Markov model.[87] In addition to no differences in health benefits, selecting HTO as a first line of treatment saved approximately US$4200 over a patient's lifetime compared with UKA and TKA while considering complications, conversions, and revisions as contributors to cost. The authors attempted to account for uncertainty in their results by rerunning their model with other potential variable values and showed that HTO was the most cost-effective intervention 57% of the time at a given willingness-to-pay value (US$50,000).[85] They concluded that HTO was the most cost-effective intervention for patients 50 to 60 years of age when compared with UKA and TKA and can delay the need for a TKA by more than a decade.[85] However, statistical uncertainty in their results prevents the complete dismissal of UKA or TKA as other viable treatments.

Similarly, Smith and colleagues[84] (2017) evaluated the lifetime cost-effectiveness of HTO, UKA, and TKA for medial tibiofemoral knee OA from the payer perspective using a Markov model, but for various age cohorts (ie, 40, 50, 60, and 70 years). Results showed that HTO was the most cost-effective treatment for middle-aged adults (ie, the 40- and 50-year-old cohorts) when compared with UKA and TKA, and UKA was more cost effective in older adults (ie, the 60- and 70-year-old cohorts). The authors attempted to account for uncertainty in their results through sensitivity analyses that demonstrated the probability HTO was cost-effective were 36% and 35% of the time at 40 and 50 years, respectively, the highest of the 3 interventions studied.[84] However, the cost effectiveness of HTO was sensitive to changes in intervention utility measures used in the model, intervention costs, and changes in the risk of revision probabilities.

According to the available literature, HTO is a viable, cost-effective treatment for young patients (<60 years of age) with medial tibiofemoral knee OA. However, stronger cost-effectiveness studies and randomized, controlled trials studying HTO are required, because there remains uncertainty in the reported modeling study results. Additionally, a limitation with the current literature is the omission of indirect costs (eg, time off employment) in cost-effectiveness analyses, which account for upwards of 80% of the overall costs for patients with knee OA.[88] Primeau and colleagues[89] evaluated HTO from a societal perspective using a within-procedure comparison that included both direct and indirect costs. They found that the study results vary depending on the costing perspective analyzed and recommend that future analyses that compare HTO with other interventions (both nonoperative and operative) should account for indirect costs.

SUMMARY

Observational studies suggest that HTO can substantially improve outcome measures important to knee joint structure and function, patient quality of life, and health care systems. We encourage HTO surgeons to establish teams of investigators with the transdisciplinary expertise necessary to conduct future comparative effectiveness studies (prospective cohort studies and randomized trials) that incorporate similar outcome measures in more rigorous clinical research designs. Although these studies are considerably more challenging, they are both warranted and required for HTO to have greater impact.

ACKNOWLEDGMENTS

The authors would like to thank all of the patients that contributed to the data presented and to the trainees involved with data collection in the laboratory. Specifically, the authors would like to thank Dr Kristyn Leitch and Dr Rebecca Moyer for grouping the data presented in figures.

REFERENCES

1. Spahn G, Hofmann GO, von Engelhardt LV, et al. The impact of a high tibial valgus osteotomy and unicondylar medial arthroplasty on the treatment for knee osteoarthritis: a meta-analysis. Knee Surg Sports Traumatol Arthrosc 2013;21(1):96–112.
2. Birmingham TB, Moyer R, Leitch K, et al. Changes in biomechanical risk factors for knee osteoarthritis and their association with 5-year clinically important improvement after limb realignment surgery. Osteoarthritis Cartilage 2017; 25(12):1999–2006.
3. Giffin JR, Shannon FJ. The role of the high tibial osteotomy in the unstable knee. Sports Med Arthrosc Rev 2007;15(1):23–31.
4. Lee OS, Ahn S, Ahn JH, et al. Effectiveness of concurrent procedures during high tibial osteotomy for medial compartment osteoarthritis: a systematic review and meta-analysis. Arch Orthop Trauma Surg 2018;138(2):227–36.
5. W-Dahl A, Robertsson O, Lohmander LS. High tibial osteotomy in Sweden, 1998-2007: a population-based study of the use and rate of revision to knee arthroplasty. Acta Orthop 2012;83(3):244–8.
6. Wright J, Heck D, Hawker G, et al. Rates of tibial osteotomies in Canada and the United States. Clin Orthop Relat Res 1995;(319):266–75.
7. Khoshbin A, Sheth U, Ogilvie-Harris D, et al. The effect of patient, provider and surgical factors on survivorship of high tibial osteotomy to total knee arthroplasty:

a population-based study. Knee Surg Sports Traumatol Arthrosc 2017;25(3): 887–94.

8. Brouwer RW, Huizinga MR, Duivenvoorden T, et al. Osteotomy for treating knee osteoarthritis. Cochrane Database Syst Rev 2014;(12):CD004019.

9. Brown GA. AAOS clinical practice guideline: treatment of osteoarthritis of the knee: evidence-based guideline, 2nd edition. J Am Acad Orthop Surg 2013; 21(9):577–9.

10. Wright JG, Swiontkowski MF, Heckman JD. Introducing levels of evidence to the journal. J Bone Joint Surg Am 2003;85-A(1):1–3.

11. Leitch KM, Birmingham TB, Dunning CE, et al. Medial opening wedge high tibial osteotomy alters knee moments in multiple planes during walking and stair ascent. Gait Posture 2015;42(2):165–71.

12. Marriott K, Birmingham TB, Kean CO, et al. Five-year changes in gait biomechanics after concomitant high tibial osteotomy and ACL reconstruction in patients with medial knee osteoarthritis. Am J Sports Med 2015;43(9):2277–85.

13. Takemae T, Omori G, Nishino K, et al. Three-dimensional knee motion before and after high tibial osteotomy for medial knee osteoarthritis. J Orthop Sci 2006;11(6): 601–6.

14. Collins B, Getgood A, Alomar AZ, et al. A case series of lateral opening wedge high tibial osteotomy for valgus malalignment. Knee Surg Sports Traumatol Arthrosc 2013;21(1):152–60.

15. Lee SH, Lee OS, Teo SH, et al. Change in gait after high tibial osteotomy: a systematic review and meta-analysis. Gait Posture 2017;57:57–68.

16. Sischek EL, Birmingham TB, Leitch KM, et al. Staged medial opening wedge high tibial osteotomy for bilateral varus gonarthrosis: biomechanical and clinical outcomes. Knee Surg Sports Traumatol Arthrosc 2014;22(11):2672–81.

17. Moyer RF, Birmingham TB, Dombroski CE, et al. Combined effects of a valgus knee brace and lateral wedge foot orthotic on the external knee adduction moment in patients with varus gonarthrosis. Arch Phys Med Rehabil 2013; 94(1):103–12.

18. Briem K, Ramsey DK, Newcomb W, et al. Effects of the amount of valgus correction for medial compartment knee osteoarthritis on clinical outcome, knee kinetics and muscle co-contraction after opening wedge high tibial osteotomy. J Orthop Res 2007;25(3):311–8.

19. Prodromos CC, Andriacchi TP, Galante JO. A relationship between gait and clinical changes following high tibial osteotomy. J Bone Joint Surg Am 1985;67(8): 1188–94.

20. Komistek RD, Dennis DA, Northcut EJ, et al. An in vivo analysis of the effectiveness of the osteoarthritic knee brace during heel-strike of gait. J Arthroplasty 1999;14(6):738–42.

21. Salim R, Salzler MJ, Bergin MA, et al. Fluoroscopic determination of the tibial insertion of the posterior cruciate ligament in the sagittal plane. Am J Sports Med 2015;43(5):1142–6.

22. Miyazaki T, Wada M, Kawahara H, et al. Dynamic load at baseline can predict radiographic disease progression in medial compartment knee osteoarthritis. Ann Rheum Dis 2002;61(7):617–22.

23. Ramsey DK, Snyder-Mackler L, Lewek M, et al. Effect of anatomic realignment on muscle function during gait in patients with medial compartment knee osteoarthritis. Arthritis Rheum 2007;57(3):389–97.

24. Kean CO, Birmingham TB, Garland SJ, et al. Preoperative strength training for patients undergoing high tibial osteotomy: a prospective cohort study with historical controls. J Orthop Sports Phys Ther 2011;41(2):52–9.
25. Niemeyer P, Koestler W, Kaehny C, et al. Two-year results of open-wedge high tibial osteotomy with fixation by medial plate fixator for medial compartment arthritis with varus malalignment of the knee. Arthroscopy 2008;24(7):796–804.
26. Kawazoe T, Takahashi T. Recovery of muscle strength after high tibial osteotomy. J Orthop Sci 2003;8(2):160–5.
27. Machner A, Pap G, Krohn A, et al. Quadriceps muscle function after high tibial osteotomy for osteoarthritis of the knee. Clin Orthop Relat Res 2002;399:177–83.
28. Kanamiya T, Naito M, Hara M, et al. The influences of biomechanical factors on cartilage regeneration after high tibial osteotomy for knees with medial compartment osteoarthritis: clinical and arthroscopic observations. Arthroscopy 2002; 18(7):725–9.
29. Koshino T, Wada S, Ara Y, et al. Regeneration of degenerated articular cartilage after high tibial valgus osteotomy for medial compartmental osteoarthritis of the knee. Knee 2003;10(3):229–36.
30. Jung WH, Takeuchi R, Chun CW, et al. Second-look arthroscopic assessment of cartilage regeneration after medial opening-wedge high tibial osteotomy. Arthroscopy 2014;30(1):72–9.
31. Le Graverand MP, Buck RJ, Wyman BT, et al. Change in regional cartilage morphology and joint space width in osteoarthritis participants versus healthy controls: a multicentre study using 3.0 Tesla MRI and Lyon-Schuss radiography. Ann Rheum Dis 2010;69(1):155–62.
32. Moyer R, Birmingham T, Lorbergs A, et al. Decreased medial compartment loading and increased medial femorotibial articular cartilage thickness 12 months after limb realignment surgery. Osteoarthritis Cartilage 2018;26:S279–80.
33. Rutgers M, Bartels LW, Tsuchida AI, et al. Dgemric as a tool for measuring changes in cartilage quality following high tibial osteotomy: a feasibility study. Osteoarthritis Cartilage 2012;20(10):1134–41.
34. Besselink NJ, Vincken KL, Bartels LW, et al. Cartilage quality (Dgemric Index) following knee joint distraction or high tibial osteotomy. Cartilage 2018. https://doi.org/10.1177/1947603518777578. 1947603518777578.
35. Parker DA, Beatty KT, Giuffre B, et al. Articular cartilage changes in patients with osteoarthritis after osteotomy. Am J Sports Med 2011;39(5):1039–45.
36. Mucha A, Dordevic M, Hirschmann A, et al. Effect of high tibial osteotomy on joint loading in symptomatic patients with varus aligned knees: a study using SPECT/CT. Knee Surg Sports Traumatol Arthrosc 2015;23(8):2315–23.
37. Gersing AS, Jungmann PM, Schwaiger BJ, et al. Longitudinal changes in subchondral bone structure as assessed with MRI are associated with functional outcome after high tibial osteotomy. J ISAKOS 2018;3(4):205–12.
38. Kraus VB, Collins JE, Hargrove D, et al. Predictive validity of biochemical biomarkers in knee osteoarthritis: data from the FNIH OA biomarkers consortium. Ann Rheum Dis 2017;76(1):186–95.
39. Guilak F, Fermor B, Keefe FJ, et al. The role of biomechanics and inflammation in cartilage injury and repair. Clin Orthop Relat Res 2004;(423):17–26.
40. Nguyen QT, Jacobsen TD, Chahine NO. Effects of inflammation on multiscale biomechanical properties of cartilaginous cells and tissues. ACS Biomater Sci Eng 2017;3(11):2644–56.
41. Berenbaum F. Osteoarthritis as an inflammatory disease (osteoarthritis is not osteoarthrosis!). Osteoarthritis Cartilage 2013;21(1):16–21.

42. McNamara IR, Birmingham TB, Marsh JD, et al. A preference-based single-item measure of quality of life following medial opening wedge high tibial osteotomy: large improvements similar to arthroplasty. Knee 2014;21(2):456–61.

43. Birmingham TB, Giffin JR, Chesworth BM, et al. Medial opening wedge high tibial osteotomy: a prospective cohort study of gait, radiographic, and patient-reported outcomes. Arthritis Rheum 2009;61(5):648–57.

44. Coventry MB, Ilstrup DM, Wallrichs SL. Proximal tibial osteotomy. a critical long-term study of eighty-seven cases. J Bone Joint Surg Am 1993;75(2):196–201.

45. Adili A, Bhandari M, Giffin R, et al. Valgus high tibial osteotomy. comparison between an Ilizarov and a Coventry wedge technique for the treatment of medial compartment osteoarthritis of the knee. Knee Surg Sports Traumatol Arthrosc 2002;10(3):169–76.

46. Akizuki S, Shibakawa A, Takizawa T, et al. The long-term outcome of high tibial osteotomy: a ten- to 20-year follow-up. J Bone Joint Surg Br 2008;90(5):592–6.

47. Borjesson M, Weidenhielm L, Mattsson E, et al. Gait and clinical measurements in patients with knee osteoarthritis after surgery: a prospective 5-year follow-up study. Knee 2005;12(2):121–7.

48. Magyar G, Toksvig-Larsen S, Lindstrand A. Hemicallotasis open-wedge osteotomy for osteoarthritis of the knee. complications in 308 operations. J Bone Joint Surg Br 1999;81(3):449–51.

49. Stukenborg-Colsman C, Wirth CJ, Lazovic D, et al. High tibial osteotomy versus unicompartmental joint replacement in unicompartmental knee joint osteoarthritis: 7-10-year follow-up prospective randomised study. Knee 2001;8(3):187–94.

50. Floerkemeier S, Staubli AE, Schroeter S, et al. Outcome after high tibial open-wedge osteotomy: a retrospective evaluation of 533 patients. Knee Surg Sports Traumatol Arthrosc 2013;21(1):170–80.

51. DeMeo PJ, Johnson EM, Chiang PP, et al. Midterm follow-up of opening-wedge high tibial osteotomy. Am J Sports Med 2010;38(10):2077–84.

52. Hoorntje A, Witjes S, Kuijer P, et al. High rates of return to sports activities and work after osteotomies around the knee: a systematic review and meta-analysis. Sports Med 2017;47(11):2219–44.

53. Bode G, von Heyden J, Pestka J, et al. Prospective 5-year survival rate data following open-wedge valgus high tibial osteotomy. Knee Surg Sports Traumatol Arthrosc 2015;23(7):1949–55.

54. Faschingbauer M, Nelitz M, Urlaub S, et al. Return to work and sporting activities after high tibial osteotomy. Int Orthop 2015;39(8):1527–34.

55. Saier T, Minzlaff P, Feucht MJ, et al. Health-related quality of life after open-wedge high tibial osteotomy. Knee Surg Sports Traumatol Arthrosc 2017;25(3):934–42.

56. Schroter S, Mueller J, van Heerwaarden R, et al. Return to work and clinical outcome after open wedge HTO. Knee Surg Sports Traumatol Arthrosc 2013;21(1):213–9.

57. Hernigou P, Queinnec S, Picard L, et al. Safety of a novel high tibial osteotomy locked plate fixation for immediate full weight-bearing: a case-control study. Int Orthop 2013;37(12):2377–84.

58. Asik M, Sen C, Kilic B, et al. High tibial osteotomy with puddu plate for the treatment of varus gonarthrosis. Knee Surg Sports Traumatol Arthrosc 2006;14(10):948–54.

59. Lobenhoffer P, Agneskirchner JD. Improvements in Surgical Technique of Valgus High Tibial Osteotomy. Knee Surg Sports Traumatol Arthrosc 2003;11(3):132–8.

60. Ihle C, Ateschrang A, Grunwald L, et al. Health-related quality of life and clinical outcomes following medial open wedge high tibial osteotomy: a prospective study. BMC Musculoskelet Disord 2016;17:215.

61. Gstottner M, Pedross F, Liebensteiner M, et al. Long-term outcome after high tibial osteotomy. Arch Orthop Trauma Surg 2008;128(1):111–5.

62. Bonasia DE, Dettoni F, Sito G, et al. Medial opening wedge high tibial osteotomy for medial compartment overload/arthritis in the varus knee: prognostic factors. Am J Sports Med 2014;42(3):690–8.

63. Altay MA, Erturk C, Altay N, et al. Clinical and radiographic outcomes of medial open-wedge high tibial osteotomy with Anthony-K plate: prospective minimum five year follow-up data. Int Orthop 2016;40(7):1447–54.

64. Niinimaki TT, Eskelinen A, Mann BS, et al. Survivorship of high tibial osteotomy in the treatment of osteoarthritis of the knee: Finnish registry-based study of 3195 knees. J Bone Joint Surg Br 2012;94(11):1517–21.

65. Polat G, Balci HI, Cakmak MF, et al. Long-term results and comparison of the three different high tibial osteotomy and fixation techniques in medial compartment arthrosis. J Orthop Surg Res 2017;12(1):44.

66. Kim JH, Kim HJ, Lee DH. Survival of opening versus closing wedge high tibial osteotomy: a meta-analysis. Sci Rep 2017;7(1):7296.

67. Bonasia DE, Governale G, Spolaore S, et al. High tibial osteotomy. Curr Rev Musculoskelet Med 2014;7(4):292–301.

68. Naudie D, Bourne RB, Rorabeck CH, et al. The Install Award. survivorship of the high tibial valgus osteotomy. a 10- to -22-year followup study. Clin Orthop Relat Res 1999;(367):18–27.

69. Schallberger A, Jacobi M, Wahl P, et al. High tibial valgus osteotomy in unicompartmental medial osteoarthritis of the knee: a retrospective follow-up study over 13-21 years. Knee Surg Sports Traumatol Arthrosc 2011;19(1):122–7.

70. Koshino T, Yoshida T, Ara Y, et al. Fifteen to twenty-eight years' follow-up results of high tibial valgus osteotomy for osteoarthritic knee. Knee 2004;11(6):439–44.

71. Ekeland A, Nerhus TK, Dimmen S, et al. Good functional results following high tibial opening-wedge osteotomy of knees with medial osteoarthritis: a prospective study with a mean of 8.3years of follow-up. Knee 2017;24(2):380–9.

72. Duivenvoorden T, van Diggele P, Reijman M, et al. Adverse events and survival after closing- and opening-wedge high tibial osteotomy: a comparative study of 412 patients. Knee Surg Sports Traumatol Arthrosc 2017;25(3):895–901.

73. Dean CS, Liechti DJ, Chahla J, et al. Clinical outcomes of high tibial osteotomy for knee instability: a systematic review. Orthop J Sports Med 2016;4(3). 2325967116633419.

74. Spahn G. Complications in high tibial (medial opening wedge) osteotomy. Arch Orthop Trauma Surg 2004;124(10):649–53.

75. Schroter S, Gonser CE, Konstantinidis L, et al. High complication rate after biplanar open wedge high tibial osteotomy stabilized with a new spacer plate (position HTO plate) without bone substitute. Arthroscopy 2011;27(5):644–52.

76. Martin R, Birmingham TB, Willits K, et al. Adverse event rates and classifications in medial opening wedge high tibial osteotomy. Am J Sports Med 2014;42(5): 1118–26.

77. Warden SJ, Morris HG, Crossley KM, et al. Delayed- and non-union following opening wedge high tibial osteotomy: surgeons' results from 182 completed cases. Knee Surg Sports Traumatol Arthrosc 2005;13(1):34–7.

78. Woodacre T, Ricketts M, Evans JT, et al. Complications associated with opening wedge high tibial osteotomy - a review of the literature and of 15 years of experience. Knee 2016;23(2):276–82.
79. Duivenvoorden T, Brouwer RW, Baan A, et al. Comparison of closing-wedge and opening-wedge high tibial osteotomy for medial compartment osteoarthritis of the knee: a randomized controlled trial with a six-year follow-up. J Bone Joint Surg Am 2014;96(17):1425–32.
80. van den Bekerom MP, Patt TW, Kleinhout MY, et al. Early complications after high tibial osteotomy: a comparison of two techniques. J Knee Surg 2008;21(1):68–74.
81. Miller BS, Downie B, McDonough EB, et al. Complications after medial opening wedge high tibial osteotomy. Arthroscopy 2009;25(6):639–46.
82. Gaasbeek RD, Nicolaas L, Rijnberg WJ, et al. Correction accuracy and collateral laxity in open versus closed wedge high tibial osteotomy. a one-year randomised controlled study. Int Orthop 2010;34(2):201–7.
83. Song EK, Seon JK, Park SJ, et al. The complications of high tibial osteotomy: closing- versus opening-wedge methods. J Bone Joint Surg Br 2010;92(9): 1245–52.
84. Smith WB 2nd, Steinberg J, Scholtes S, et al. Medial compartment knee osteoarthritis: age-stratified cost-effectiveness of total knee arthroplasty, unicompartmental knee arthroplasty, and high tibial osteotomy. Knee Surg Sports Traumatol Arthrosc 2017;25(3):924–33.
85. Konopka JF, Gomoll AH, Thornhill TS, et al. The cost-effectiveness of surgical treatment of medial unicompartmental knee osteoarthritis in younger patients: a computer model-based evaluation. J Bone Joint Surg Am 2015;97(10):807–17.
86. Drummond MF, Sculpher MJ, Torrance GW, et al. Methods for the economic evaluation of health care programme. 3rd edition. Oxford (England): Oxford University Press; 2005.
87. Briggs A, Sculpher M. An introduction to Markov modelling for economic evaluation. Pharmacoeconomics 1998;13(4):397–409.
88. Gupta S, Hawker GA, Laporte A, et al. The economic burden of disabling hip and knee osteoarthritis (OA) from the perspective of individuals living with this condition. Rheumatology (Oxford) 2005;44(12):1531–7.
89. Primeau CA, Marsh JD, Birmingham TB, et al. The importance of costing perspective: an example evaluating cost-effectiveness of a locking versus non-locking plate in medial opening wedge high tibial osteotomy. Can J Surg 2019; 62(1):E14–6.
90. Peterfy CG, Schneider E, Nevitt M. The osteoarthritis initiative: report on the design rationale for the magnetic resonance imaging protocol for the knee. Osteoarthritis Cartilage 2008;16(12):1433–41.

Medial Opening-Wedge High Tibial Osteotomy for Medial Compartment Arthrosis/Overload

Molly Day, MD, ATC[a],*, Brian R. Wolf, MD, MS[b]

KEYWORDS

- Medial opening-wedge high tibial osteotomy • Medial tibiofemoral osteoarthrosis
- Medial tibiofemoral compartment overload • Varus deformity • Mechanical axis

KEY POINTS

- The goal of medial opening-wedge high tibial osteotomy is to correct limb malalignment and transfer weightbearing from the degenerated medial compartment to the unaffected lateral compartment.
- Indications include medial compartment knee arthrosis or overload associated with varus alignment, with or without instability or osteochondral defects requiring resurfacing.
- Ideal patient characteristics include age younger than 55 to 60 years, normal weight, preserved range of motion, and isolated medial compartment osteoarthritis or overload.
- Complications include overcorrection, undercorrection, fracture of the lateral tibial cortex with proximal fragment instability, joint contracture, infection, compartment syndrome, nonunion or delayed union, deep venous thrombosis, neurovascular injury, and loss of fixation.
- In appropriate patients, medial opening-wedge high tibial osteotomy produces good outcomes.

Disclosures: Dr B.R. Wolf reports the following disclosures: AAOS: Board or committee member; American Orthopedic Society for Sports Medicine: Board or committee member; Arthrex, Inc: Other financial or material support; CONMED Linvatec: Paid consultant; Mid America Orthopedic Association: Board or committee member; Orthopaedic Research and Education Foundation (OREF), United States: Research support; Orthopedic Journal of Sports Medicine: Editorial or governing board; Smith and Nephew: Other financial or material support.

[a] Department of Orthopedics and Rehabilitation, University of Iowa Hospitals and Clinics, 200 Hawkins Drive, Iowa City, IA 52242, USA; [b] Department of Orthopedics and Rehabilitation, University of Iowa Hospitals and Clinics, University of Iowa Athletics, 2701 Prairie Meadow Drive, Iowa City, IA 52240, USA
* Corresponding author.
E-mail address: molly-day@uiowa.edu

Clin Sports Med 38 (2019) 331–349
https://doi.org/10.1016/j.csm.2019.02.003
0278-5919/19/© 2019 Elsevier Inc. All rights reserved.

sportsmed.theclinics.com

INTRODUCTION

Medial knee osteoarthritis is common and can be a clinical challenge, especially for young, active patients who are not ideal candidates for arthroplasty. High tibial osteotomy (HTO) was developed to transfer the mechanical axis to decrease load and delay the progression of osteoarthritis.[1,2] Evidence has shown that offloading the medial knee compartment can lead to symptomatic improvement and cartilage regeneration.[3,4] In 1961, Jackson and Waugh[5] first reported HTO to treat medial knee osteoarthritis. However, HTO did not become popular until Coventry[6] in 1965 promoted HTO as a treatment for medial compartment arthritis with varus deformity. Since then, the procedure has seen drastic improvements in technique, fixation, and patient selection in recent years, with fewer complications.

Several correction osteotomy techniques exist for unicompartmental knee osteoarthritis, including lateral closing wedge, medial opening-wedge, dome osteotomies, and Ilizarov or external fixator techniques. The focus of this article is to describe and review the surgical technique for medial opening-wedge HTO for patients with medial compartment arthrosis or overload, and discuss the complications and outcomes. In appropriately indicated patients, medial opening-wedge HTO is widely accepted to produce good outcomes for younger, active patients with symptomatic medial compartment osteoarthrosis.[7–10] There are a variety of surgical techniques described for medial opening-wedge HTO, including a variety of methods of osteotomy fixation, grafting, and concomitant procedures. Graft choices include autograft (generally iliac crest), allograft, or osteoconductive synthetic bone graft substitute. The authors prefer to use wedges fashioned out of a femoral head allograft to avoid donor site morbidity, maintain the ability to fill a wedge-shaped HTO defect with fashioned bone wedges, and a shorter surgical time compared with autograft harvest.

Medial opening-wedge osteotomy is the senior author's preferred technique for HTO. There are several advantages of medial opening-wedge osteotomy compared with the traditional lateral closed-wedge alternative. First, there is more precision and the ability to achieve predictable correction in the coronal and sagittal planes, as the medial opening can be "dialed in" and progressively assessed in the operating room. The opening can be increased or decreased as needed to achieve the appropriate correction. Next, medial opening-wedge HTO avoids the need for proximal tibiofibular joint disruption or proximal fibula osteotomy, and thus almost eliminates the risk of peroneal nerve injury. Last, medial opening-wedge HTO preserves tibial bone and theoretically leads to easier conversion to total knee arthroplasty (TKA) if needed in the future.[11]

The disadvantages of medial opening-wedge HTO are the creation of a defect with the need for bone grafting, risk of nonunion, and possible loss of correction owing to collapse or instability of the construct.[12] In the instance of large corrections (>15.0–17.5 mm of opening), medial opening-wedge osteotomy may not be the ideal method of axis correction given the larger risk for nonunion, with a greater risk for nonunion in corrections with greater than 15.0 to 17.5 mm of opening as compared with closing-wedge or external fixation/Ilizarov techniques. Additionally, depending on the hardware construct used for fixation, there are often more postoperative restrictions and a longer period of nonweightbearing or restricted weightbearing after surgery. In addition, extra attention should be given to the slope, because most medial opening-wedge HTO techniques and systems have the potential to inadvertently increase tibial sagittal slope.

INDICATIONS

The main indications for medial opening-wedge HTO include varus knee alignment associated with (1) medial compartment osteoarthritis in a stable knee, (2) medial compartment osteoarthritis with associated knee instability (eg, anterior cruciate ligament, posterior cruciate ligament, lateral collateral ligament, or combined deficiencies), (3) painful medial compartment with associated medial meniscus deficiency, or (4) concomitant osteochondral lesions or defects requiring resurfacing procedures. Patients have often failed nonsurgical management using a combination of nonpharmacologic and pharmacologic treatments.

The ideal patients are physiologically young (younger than 55–60 years), with isolated medial compartment disease, an absence of lateral tibial thrust, and a preserved range of motion, with less than 15° of anatomic varus angulation.[7,13,14] Relative contraindications include patients older than 65 years, severe, end-stage osteoarthritis in the medial compartment, tricompartmental osteoarthritis, inflammatory knee arthritis, loss of range of motion (<120°) and/or flexion contracture of greater than 5°, smoking status, and a high body mass index (>30).[7,13]

PREOPERATIVE PLANNING

Preoperative planning is essential to achieve good results for HTO, and begins with a detailed history and physical examination, along with appropriate imaging. Significant aspects of the patient's history should include previous injury and all prior treatment and/or surgical procedures to the extremity and history of mechanical symptoms, which may indicate the need for arthroscopic intervention. Physical examination features should include a patient's gait and stance, patellar tracking, range of motion, and ligamentous stability. Limb length discrepancy, ankle deformity, and instability should also be determined and considered before surgery.

Essential radiographs that are critical for preoperative planning include standing (weightbearing) bilateral anteroposterior long leg films (**Fig. 1**), anteroposterior, lateral and merchant (axial) views of the knee. Other views to consider include the 45° flexed weight-bearing posteroanterior view, and valgus or varus stress views. It is important to identify whether the lateral joint space width is maintained in valgus-stress knee radiographs, because the postoperative weightbearing portion becomes the lateral compartment. It is also important to evaluate need for concomitant procedures, such as arthroscopy, cartilage resurfacing, and/or ligamentous reconstruction. Therefore, MRI may be considered to further evaluate cartilage, menisci, and ligaments.

Radiographic Templating

The goal of radiographic templating is to determine the desired location and direction of the osteotomy line, and the desired angle of correction. In a varus knee with medial compartment osteoarthritis, best results are achieved when the anatomic axis is corrected to 8° to 10° valgus.[15] This has also been described as when the weightbearing line passes through the lateral plateau at 62% to 66% of its width.[16]

To determine the mechanical axis on a full-length, standing anteroposterior radiograph, draw a line from the center of the femoral head to the center of the tibiotalar joint (**Fig. 2**). Next, draw a line from the center of the femoral head to the desired new point of axis in the lateral compartment, and from the center of the tibiotalar joint to the same point in the lateral knee (**Fig. 3**). The degree of correction required is determined by the angle formed by the intersection of lines from the hip and ankle (**Fig. 4**). Measure the width of the tibia at the HTO site, as well as the same distance along

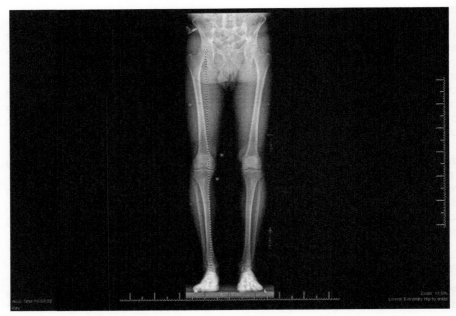

Fig. 1. Standing (weightbearing) bilateral anteroposterior long leg radiograph.

crossing lines. The amount of opening-wedge is equal to the angle at the measured distance (**Fig. 5**).

SURGICAL TECHNIQUE

1. The patient is placed supine on a radiolucent operating table with a bump as needed to place the involved lower extremity in neutral position. It is critical that the patient is positioned on a table that allows fluoroscopy of the entire lower extremity, including the hip joint. A tourniquet is placed on the upper thigh. Bony anatomic landmarks, including the patellar tendon, tibial tuberosity, joint line, and Gerdy's tubercle are marked with a surgical marking pen.
2. When indicated, arthroscopic surgery is performed to treat associated injuries. This can include chondroplasty, microfracture, or other cartilage restoration procedures if a focal cartilage defect is present in the medial compartment. Arthroscopy can also confirm the integrity of the lateral compartment before HTO.
3. An approximately 5-cm longitudinal incision is made between the medial border of the tibial tubercle and posteromedial border of the tibia from the inferior patella to 3 cm distal to the tibial tuberosity.
4. The incision is carried through the skin and dissection proceeds through the subcutaneous tissue with a combination of a sharp knife and electrocautery, until the anterior aspect of the proximal tibial and sartorial fascia are exposed.
5. The sartorial fascia is longitudinally incised using an inverted, L-shaped incision through the periosteum, and the insertions of the pes anserinus, gracilis, and semitendinosus are retracted or detached (**Fig. 6**). The superficial layer of the medial collateral ligament is then elevated posteriorly subperiosteally using electrocautery and a Cobb elevator. Surgeons should aim to elevate this tissue in a thick sleeve to allow repair over the osteotomy site at the end of the case.

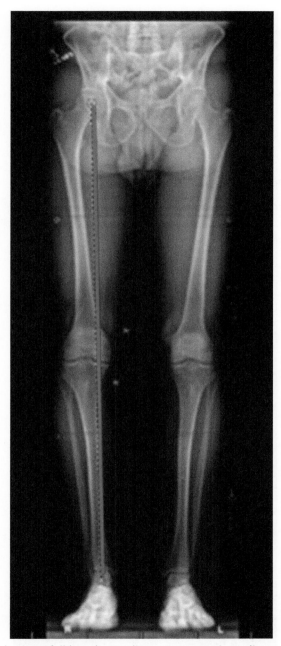

Fig. 2. Mechanical axis on full-length, standing anteroposterior radiograph.

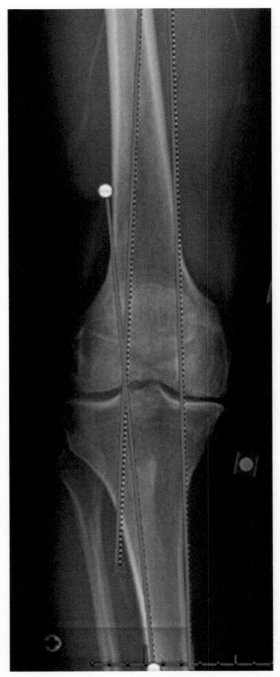

Fig. 3. Lines from center of femoral head to desired point of axis on lateral knee joint, and from the center of the tibiotalar joint to the same point in the lateral knee.

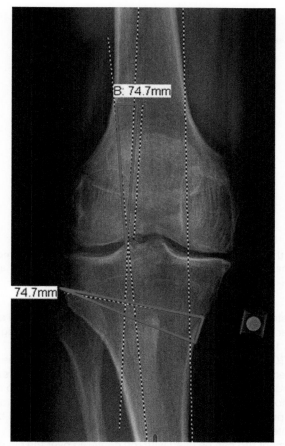

Fig. 4. Degree of osteotomy correction required, determined by the angle formed by the intersection of lines from the hip and ankle.

6. The tissue of the posteromedial tibia is elevated and a blunt radiolucent retractor is placed around the posteromedial proximal tibia along the posterior cortex to protect the posterior neurovascular structures (**Fig. 7**).

7. The tibial tubercle and medial border of the patellar tendon are then identified. The osteotomy should be carried out immediately proximal to the tuberosity. The patellar tendon is retracted anteriorly and laterally and protected throughout the procedure.

8. Using fluoroscopy, 2 to 3 guidewires are inserted in parallel fashion at the medial cortex 2 mm proximal and parallel to the HTO site, near the medial metaphyseal flare of the tibia, which is approximately 4 cm distal from the joint line. The pins are directed parallel to the proximal tibiofibular joint, creating an osteotomy plane (**Fig. 8**). The cut should be aimed toward the tip of the fibular head, approximately 1.5 cm below the lateral articular surface (**Fig. 9**). The osteotomy should be parallel to the tibial slope, so care should be taken to follow the patient's natural posterior tibial slope, which is approximately 10°.

9. With retractors protecting the soft tissue anteriorly and posteriorly, the medial and anterior cortical cut is made along the guide pins using a small, oscillating bone

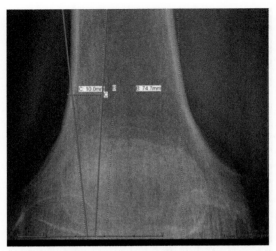

Fig. 5. Width of the tibia measured at the HTO site, as well as the same distance along crossing lines. The amount of opening-wedge is equal to the angle at the measured distance.

    saw. Thin osteotomes are then used below the pins to open and advance the osteotomy laterally to within 1 cm of the lateral tibial cortex, leaving a 10-mm bony hinge (**Figs. 10** and **11**).

10. Once the HTO is mobile, calibrated wedges are inserted into the osteotomy site and advanced until the desired opening is achieved (**Fig. 12**). This process should be performed slowly and carefully with the use of fluoroscopy to avoid extension of the osteotomy proximally into the joint or laterally. Significant fracturing laterally can lead to proximal fragment instability, so fluoroscopy should be monitored to ensure no lateral displacement or instability occurs.

11. A long alignment rod can be used with rod centered over the hip and ankle. In his position, the rod should cross the knee at approximately 62% to 66% of the proximal tibial width (**Fig. 13**).

12. The anatomic tibial slope should be assessed using fluoroscopy before final fixation. The tendency is to inadvertently increase the slope, so the orientation of the

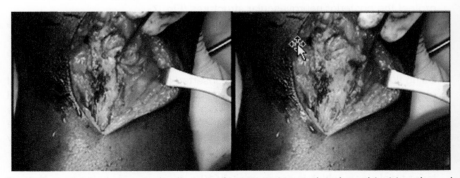

Fig. 6. Sartorial fascia longitudinally incised using an inverted, L-shaped incision through the periosteum. The insertions of the pes anserinus, the gracilis, and the semitendinosus are retracted or detached.

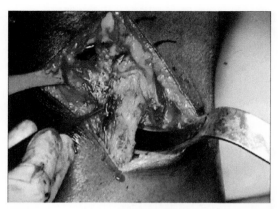

Fig. 7. Elevated tissue of the posteromedial tibia, with a blunt retractor placed around the posteromedial proximal tibia along the posterior cortex to protect the posterior neurovascular structures.

tibial articular surface in the sagittal plane should be carefully evaluated. In some instances, increasing or decreasing the posterior tibial slope can be accomplished to address cruciate ligament deficiency, as decreasing the slope will subsequently decrease anterior tibial translate in anterior cruciate ligament-deficient patients. Similarly, increasing the tibial slope in posterior cruciate ligament deficiency will increase anterior tibial translation, assisting with knee stability. The slope can be modified by adjusting the opening-wedge anteriorly or posteriorly on the medial side. More posterior opening and less anterior opening will protect against increasing the tibial slope significantly.

13. Fixation is then performed. Authors prefer to use a 4-hole stainless steel Arthrex Puddu plate (Arthrex, Inc, Naples, FL). which includes a slightly wedged metal tooth that inserts into the HTO site. Fixation is performed using two 4.5 bicortical screws distally, taking care to not penetrate the proximal tibiofibular joint, and two 6.5 partially threaded cancellous screws proximally (**Figs. 14** and **15**).

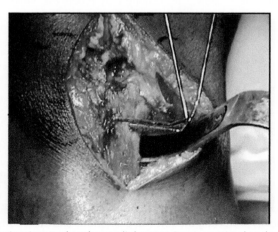

Fig. 8. Two guidewires inserted at the medial cortex 2 mm proximal and parallel to the HTO site, near the metaphyseal flare of the tibia, approximately 4 cm distal from the joint line. The pins are directed parallel to the proximal tibiofibular joint, creating an osteotomy plane.

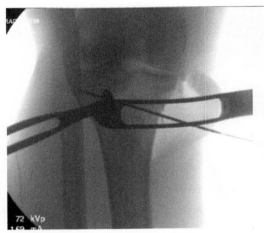

Fig. 9. Fluoroscopy image showing osteotomy cut aimed toward the tip of the fibular head, approximately 1 cm below the lateral articular surface.

14. The osteotomy gap is then filled with bone graft. Bone graft options include bone substitutes, allograft, or autograft. The senior author prefers to use allograft wedges cut from femoral head allograft (**Figs. 16** and **17**) to match the dimensions of the opening created with the HTO. Graft can be placed deep to the fixation plate, as well as anterior and posterior to completely fill the defect.
15. For closure, the surgeon can usually pull the medial collateral ligament, pes tendons, and periosteum over the majority if not all of the hardware using 0-Vicryl. This results in less hardware irritation and pain (**Fig. 18**).

POSTOPERATIVE REGIMEN

Postoperatively, the patient is fit with a hinged knee brace set at 0° to 90°, and is nonweightbearing on the operative extremity. If the patient is doing well at 6 weeks postoperatively, the patient is slowly transitioned to touch–toe weightbearing and to

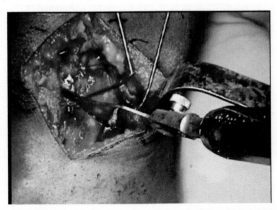

Fig. 10. With retractors protecting the soft tissue anteriorly and posteriorly, the medial and anterior cortical cut is made along the guide pins using a small, oscillating bone saw. Thin osteotomes used below the pins to open and advance the osteotomy laterally to within 1 cm of the lateral tibial cortex, leaving a 10-mm hinge.

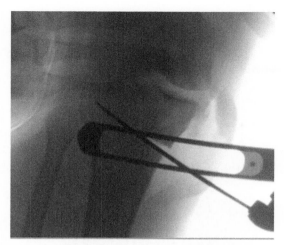

Fig. 11. Fluoroscopy imaging showing thin osteotome used below the pins to open and advance the osteotomy laterally to within 1 cm of the lateral tibial cortex, leaving a 10-mm hinge.

weightbearing as tolerated gradually over the next 4 to 6 weeks. The patient is maintained in the brace for 3 months. Radiographs are taken at 6 weeks and 3 months postoperatively to ensure healing (**Fig. 19**), and long leg alignment films are taken at 6 months postoperatively.

RESULTS

The results of HTO vary across the literature, but in general there is good evidence to show that HTO provides good relief of pain and restoration of function for medial arthrosis of the knee. Survivorship of opening and/or closing wedge HTO has been found to be 70% to 94% at 5 to 9 years, 74% to 98% at 10 years, 66% to 91% at 15 years, and 52% to 54% at 17 to 18 years.[13,15,17–20] In a systematic review by Brouwer and colleagues,[21] there is "silver level" evidence that HTO improves knee

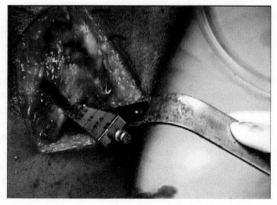

Fig. 12. Calibrated wedges inserted into the osteotomy site, advanced until the desired open is achieved.

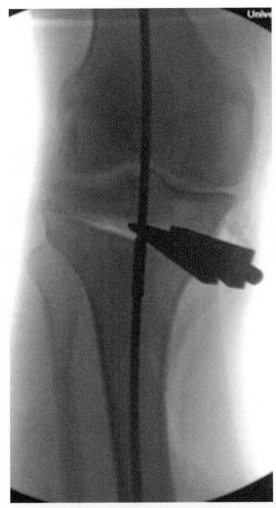

Fig. 13. Fluoroscopy image showing the long alignment rod used with rod centered over the hip and ankle. In his position, the rod should cross the knee at approximately 62% to 66% of the proximal tibial width.

function and reduces pain in patients with medial knee arthrosis. Results of HTO deteriorate over time, which has been well-accepted in the literature, and the long-term results of HTO depend on the accuracy of the correction.[15,22] In a comparison of medial opening-wedge or lateral closing-wedge HTO, a previous systematic review has shown no difference in the incidence of complications or clinical outcomes between the 2 techniques.[23] Additionally, a randomized controlled trial by Duivenvoorden and colleagues[24] did not show a difference in clinical or radiographic outcomes between closing-wedge and opening-wedge osteotomies in 92 patients at 6 years postoperative. In that study, opening-wedge osteotomy was associated with a higher rate of complications, and closing-wedge with a higher conversion rate to TKA (22% vs 8%, $P = .05$).

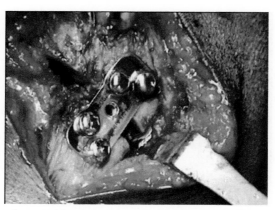

Fig. 14. A 4-hole Arthrex Puddu plate. (*Courtesy of* Arthrex, Inc, Naples, FL.)

Specific to opening-wedge HTO, there is limited literature describing long-term outcomes. In a metaanalysis with 20 years of follow-up, the survivorship at 5, 10, 15, and 20 years was 92.4%, 84.5%, 77.3%, and 72.3%, respectively.[25] Similarly, in a study with a mean follow-up of 51 months, Bonasia and colleagues[7] reported survivorship of 98.7% at 5 years and 75.9% at 7.5 years, using a Puddu plate for fixation. Bode and colleagues[26] evaluated 62 patients after HTO using TomoFix (Synthes, Solothurn, Switzerland), with a 96% survival rate at 5 years. Variables related to poor outcome were age greater than 56 years and postoperative knee flexion of less than 120°.

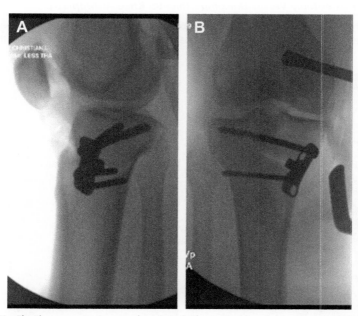

Fig. 15. (*A, B*). Fluoroscopy image showing Arthrex Puddu plate, using two 4.5 cortical screws distally and two 6.5 partially threaded cancellous screws proximally, with (*A*) lateral and (*B*) anteroposterior images.

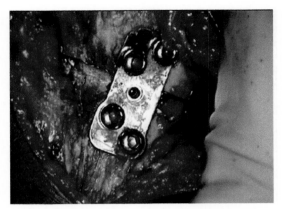

Fig. 16. Osteotomy gap filled with bone graft. Bone graft options include bone substitutes, allograft, or autograft.

Stabilization of the Osteotomy

The type or system used for fixation after opening-wedge HTO is still controversial. The most commonly used fixation devices include external fixators or plates. Comparison of the modified Puddu plate (Arthrex, Naples, FL) and the TomoFix plate (Synthes) demonstrated equal stability, but in the instance of lateral cortex fracture/instability the TomoFix plate provided superior stability.[27] Although long locking plates seems to show better biomechanical properties, hardware removal is almost always required.

High Tibial Osteotomy Versus Unicompartmental Knee Arthroplasty

Although HTO and unicompartmental knee arthroplasty (UKA) can both be performed for the treatment of unicompartmental knee osteoarthritis in young patients, there is a

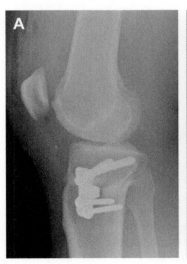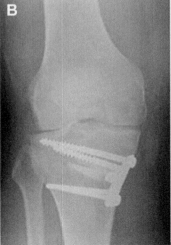

Fig. 17. Fluoroscopy image showing osteotomy gap filled with bone graft, with (A) lateral and (B) anteroposterior images.

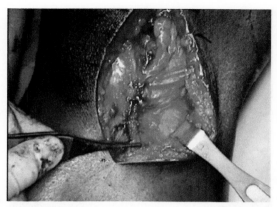

Fig. 18. The medial collateral ligament, pes tendons, and periosteum pulled over hardware using 0-Vicryl.

limited overlap of indications. Dettoni and colleagues[28] previously reported that patients who can be indicated for either HTO or UKA are active patients aged 55 to 65 years of age with 5° to 10° varus alignment, less than 5° of flexion contracture, and grade II (Ahlback) medial OA. HTO and UKA have both been shown to produce similar, satisfactory results.[21,28] HTO should be considered in younger, more active patients owing to the ability to maintain a higher level of activity without concern for accelerated wear of the arthroplasty components.

Total Knee Arthroplasty After High Tibial Osteotomy

With known deterioration after HTO, TKA represents the endpoint after failure. Performing TKA after HTO can be difficult owing to valgus alignment, scarring, and anatomic changes in the proximal tibia. Patellar height, posterior slope, and offset may influence outcomes.[21] Opening-wedge osteotomy has a potential advantage as compared with closing-wedge HTO or UKA by maintaining proximal tibia bone stock and minimizing the risk of impingement of the tibial stem to the anterior tibial cortex after conversion to TKA. In a comparison of TKA after medial opening-wedge HTO versus lateral closing-wedge HTO, there was no significant difference in clinical results or complications.[29] Furthermore, no published data have demonstrated significant differences between primary TKA and TKA after HTO.[14,30]

Complications

HTO is technically demanding and carries an established risk of complications, regardless of the technique, with reported overall complication rates of 29% to 37%.[31,32] Complications of medial opening-wedge HTO include malalignment, lateral cortex fracture (5.6%–15.6%), stiffness (1.2%), infection (4.7%–9.6%), compartment syndrome (0.9%), nonunion (0.6%–4.3%) or delayed union (2.4%–4.3%), neurovascular injury (1.7%–3.6%), deep venous thrombosis (2.3%–4.3%), hardware irritation (1.2%–7%), and loss of alignment (2.4%–15.2%).[31–35] In a study by Willey and colleagues,[36] isolated HTO or HTO with additional procedure (anterior cruciate ligament, osteoarticular transfer system [OATS], etc) showed no difference in complication rates, with complication rates of 16% to 20% for major complications and 26% to 32% for minor complications.

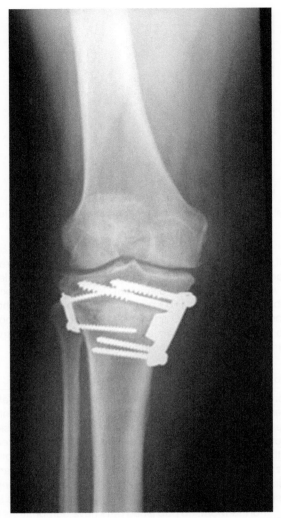

Fig. 19. Postoperative anteroposterior knee radiographs taken at 6 weeks, demonstrating healing.

Nonunion is one of the main risks in opening-wedge HTO, with an incidence ranging from 0.7% to 4.4% of patients after HTO.[34] Nonunion is increased with large corrections, smoking status, and poor fixation. Nonunion has also been associated with bone graft type, in 1 study, allograft mixed with demineralized bone matrix and/or platelet-rich plasma (PRP) was associated with increased nonunion rates.[33] Most studies with good results without bone graft used long locking plates.[37]

SUMMARY

In appropriately indicated patients, medial opening-wedge HTO is a safe and effective treatment for younger, active patients with symptomatic medial compartment osteoarthrosis associated with varus alignment. The procedure may be combined with concomitant cartilage restoration or reconstructive procedures. There are a variety of surgical techniques that exist, including various forms of fixation and use of allograft or autograft, with minimal clinically significant differences. Further studies with long-term follow-up are needed to identify ideal candidates and surgical techniques in medial opening-wedge HTO.

REFERENCES

1. Gaasbeek R, Welsing R, Barink M, et al. The influence of open and closed high tibial osteotomy on dynamic patellar tracking: a biomechanical study. Knee Surg Sports Traumatol Arthrosc 2007;15(8):978–84.
2. Aglietti P, Rinonapoli E, Stringa G, et al. Tibial osteotomy for the varus osteoarthritic knee. Clin Orthop Relat Res 1983;(176):239–51.
3. Koshino T, Wada S, Ara Y, et al. Regeneration of degenerated articular cartilage after high tibial valgus osteotomy for medial compartmental osteoarthritis of the knee. Knee 2003;10(3):229–36.
4. Jung WH, Takeuchi R, Chun CW, et al. Second-look arthroscopic assessment of cartilage regeneration after medial opening-wedge high tibial osteotomy. Arthroscopy 2014;30(1):72–9.
5. Jackson JP, Waugh W. Tibial osteotomy for osteoarthritis of the knee. J Bone Joint Surg Br 1961;43-b:746–51.
6. Coventry MB. Osteotomy of the upper portion of the tibia for degenerative arthritis of the knee. a preliminary report. J Bone Joint Surg Am 1965;47:984–90.
7. Bonasia DE, Dettoni F, Sito G, et al. Medial opening-wedge high tibial osteotomy for medial compartment overload/arthritis in the varus knee: prognostic factors. Am J Sports Med 2014;42(3):690–8.
8. Amendola A, Fowler PJ, Litchfield R, et al. Opening-wedge high tibial osteotomy using a novel technique: early results and complications. J Knee Surg 2004; 17(3):164–9.
9. Noyes FR, Barber SD, Simon R. High tibial osteotomy and ligament reconstruction in varus angulated, anterior cruciate ligament-deficient knees. A two- to seven-year follow-up study. Am J Sports Med 1993;21(1):2–12.
10. Noyes FR, Mayfield W, Barber-Westin SD, et al. Opening-wedge high tibial osteotomy: an operative technique and rehabilitation program to decrease complications and promote early union and function. Am J Sports Med 2006;34(8): 1262–73.
11. Brouwer RW, Bierma-Zeinstra SM, van Raaij TM, et al. Osteotomy for medial compartment arthritis of the knee using a closing wedge or an opening-wedge controlled by a Puddu plate. A one-year randomised, controlled study. J Bone Joint Surg Br 2006;88(11):1454–9.
12. Hankemeier S, Mommsen P, Krettek C, et al. Accuracy of high tibial osteotomy: comparison between open- and closed-wedge technique. Knee Surg Sports Traumatol Arthrosc 2010;18(10):1328–33.
13. Naudie D, Bourne RB, Rorabeck CH, et al. The Insall Award. Survivorship of the high tibial valgus osteotomy. A 10- to -22-year followup study. Clin Orthop Relat Res 1999;(367):18–27.
14. Amendola A, Bonasia DE. Results of high tibial osteotomy: review of the literature. Int Orthop 2010;34(2):155–60.
15. Coventry MB, Ilstrup DM, Wallrichs SL. Proximal tibial osteotomy. A critical long-term study of eighty-seven cases. J Bone Joint Surg Am 1993;75(2):196–201.

16. Dugdale TW, Noyes FR, Styer D. Preoperative planning for high tibial osteotomy. The effect of lateral tibiofemoral separation and tibiofemoral length. Clin Orthop Relat Res 1992;(274):248–64.
17. Papachristou G, Plessas S, Sourlas J, et al. Deterioration of long-term results following high tibial osteotomy in patients under 60 years of age. Int Orthop 2006;30(5):403–8.
18. Gstottner M, Pedross F, Liebensteiner M, et al. Long-term outcome after high tibial osteotomy. Arch Orthop Trauma Surg 2008;128(1):111–5.
19. Insall JN, Joseph DM, Msika C. High tibial osteotomy for varus gonarthrosis. A long-term follow-up study. J Bone Joint Surg Am 1984;66(7):1040–8.
20. Ivarsson I, Myrnerts R, Gillquist J. High tibial osteotomy for medial osteoarthritis of the knee. A 5 to 7 and 11 year follow-up. J Bone Joint Surg Br 1990;72(2):238–44.
21. Brouwer RW, Raaij van TM, Bierma-Zeinstra SM, et al. Osteotomy for treating knee osteoarthritis. Cochrane Database Syst Rev 2014;(12):CD004019.
22. Sprenger TR, Doerzbacher JF. Tibial osteotomy for the treatment of varus gonarthrosis. Survival and failure analysis to twenty-two years. J Bone Joint Surg Am 2003;85-a(3):469–74.
23. Smith TO, Sexton D, Mitchell P, et al. Opening- or closing-wedged high tibial osteotomy: a meta-analysis of clinical and radiological outcomes. Knee 2011;18(6):361–8.
24. Duivenvoorden T, Brouwer RW, Baan A, et al. Comparison of closing-wedge and opening-wedge high tibial osteotomy for medial compartment osteoarthritis of the knee: a randomized controlled trial with a six-year follow-up. J Bone Joint Surg Am 2014;96(17):1425–32.
25. Harris JD, McNeilan R, Siston RA, et al. Survival and clinical outcome of isolated high tibial osteotomy and combined biological knee reconstruction. Knee 2013;20(3):154–61.
26. Bode G, von Heyden J, Pestka J, et al. Prospective 5-year survival rate data following open-wedge valgus high tibial osteotomy. Knee Surg Sports Traumatol Arthrosc 2015;23(7):1949–55.
27. Stoffel K, Stachowiak G, Kuster M. Open wedge high tibial osteotomy: biomechanical investigation of the modified Arthrex Osteotomy Plate (Puddu Plate) and the TomoFix Plate. Clin Biomech (Bristol, Avon) 2004;19(9):944–50.
28. Dettoni F, Bonasia DE, Castoldi F, et al. High tibial osteotomy versus unicompartmental knee arthroplasty for medial compartment arthrosis of the knee: a review of the literature. Iowa Orthop J 2010;30:131–40.
29. Ehlinger M, D'Ambrosio A, Vie P, et al. Total knee arthroplasty after opening-versus closing-wedge high tibial osteotomy. A 135-case series with minimum 5-year follow-up. Orthop Traumatol Surg Res 2017;103(7):1035–9.
30. Amendola A, Rorabeck CH, Bourne RB, et al. Total knee arthroplasty following high tibial osteotomy for osteoarthritis. J Arthroplasty 1989;4(Suppl):S11–7.
31. Seo SS, Kim OG, Seo JH, et al. Complications and short-term outcomes of medial opening-wedge high tibial osteotomy using a locking plate for medial osteoarthritis of the knee. Knee Surg Relat Res 2016;28(4):289–96.
32. Miller BS, Downie B, McDonough EB, et al. Complications after medial opening-wedge high tibial osteotomy. Arthroscopy 2009;25(6):639–46.
33. Giuseffi SA, Replogle WH, Shelton WR. Opening-wedge high tibial osteotomy: review of 100 consecutive cases. Arthroscopy 2015;31(11):2128–37.
34. Spahn G. Complications in high tibial (medial opening-wedge) osteotomy. Arch Orthop Trauma Surg 2004;124(10):649–53.

35. Woodacre T, Ricketts M, Evans JT, et al. Complications associated with opening-wedge high tibial osteotomy–A review of the literature and of 15 years of experience. Knee 2016;23(2):276–82.
36. Willey M, Wolf BR, Kocaglu B, et al. Complications associated with realignment osteotomy of the knee performed simultaneously with additional reconstructive procedures. Iowa Orthop J 2010;30:55–60.
37. Niemeyer P, Schmal H, Hauschild O, et al. Open-wedge osteotomy using an internal plate fixator in patients with medial-compartment gonarthritis and varus malalignment: 3-year results with regard to preoperative arthroscopic and radiographic findings. Arthroscopy 2010;26(12):1607–16.

Lateral Opening Wedge Distal Femoral Osteotomy for Lateral Compartment Arthrosis/Overload

Carola Pilone, MD, Federica Rosso, MD, Umberto Cottino, MD, Roberto Rossi, MD, Davide Edoardo Bonasia, MD*

KEYWORDS

- DFO • Lateral opening wedge DFO • Valgus knee • Lateral compartment arthrosis
- Knee osteotomy

KEY POINTS

- Distal femoral osteotomy (DFO) is a valid option for the treatment of young and active patients with lateral compartment osteoarthritis/overload and valgus malalignment.
- DFO can be performed with a lateral opening wedge or a medial closing wedge technique, with similar results. The opening wedge technique is preferred in case of smaller corrections, is technically easier, but requires bone grafting and may have a higher rate of nonunion.
- A good candidate for an opening wedge DFO is a young (<65 year old) and active patient, with valgus malalignment (<20°) and isolated lateral compartment osteoarthritis. DFOs are also indicated in case of chronic medial collateral ligament deficiency and valgus malalignment, with or without medial compartment reconstruction.
- In varus-producing DFOs, a correction to neutral alignment (no overcorrection) is recommended. The osteotomy can be fixed with a spacer plate or with locking plates and generally the osteotomy gap requires bone grafting (auto/allograft or bone substitutes).

INTRODUCTION

Distal femoral osteotomy (DFO) is a valid option for the treatment of young and active patients with lateral compartment osteoarthritis and valgus malalignment.

The goals of the procedure are to reduce pain and arthritis progression and offload the lateral compartment. DFO can also be indicated in case of valgus knee with chronic medial collateral ligament (MCL) instability.

Financial Conflict of Interest: None.
Department of Orthopaedics and Traumatology, AO Ordine Mauriziano Hospital, University of Torino, Largo Turati 62, Torino 10128, Italy
* Corresponding author. Via Lamarmora 26, Torino 10128, Italy.
E-mail address: davidebonasia@virgilio.it

Clin Sports Med 38 (2019) 351–359
https://doi.org/10.1016/j.csm.2019.02.004
0278-5919/19/© 2019 Elsevier Inc. All rights reserved.

sportsmed.theclinics.com

DFOs can be performed with a lateral closing wedge (CWDFO) or a medial opening wedge (OWDFO) technique.

OWDFO is easier and more precise than CWDFO, but has a higher rate of nonunion.[1] Lateral opening wedge DFO is usually preferred for smaller corrections, whereas medial closing wedge for larger corrections and in patients with high risk of nonunion (ie, smokers).

This article is a review of the recent literature about opening wedge DFO, with particular attention to the indications, surgical technique, and outcomes.

In the past, valgus deformity of the knee was generally attributed to femoral anatomic variants: that is, lateral femoral epicondyle hypoplasia or decreased anatomic lateral distal femoral articular angle. For this reason, many investigators adopted DFO as a preferred technique to correct these deformities. However, recent studies have shown that valgus malalignment is attributable to tibial deformity in most patients and that a combined femoral- and tibial-based deformity is more common than an isolated femoral-based deformity.[2] Therefore, in theory, varus osteotomies should be performed at the tibial site or as a double-level osteotomy in a relevant number of patients to avoid an oblique joint line.[3]

INDICATIONS AND CONTRAINDICATIONS

A good candidate for a DFO is a young and active patient (<65 year old), with valgus malalignment (<20°) and isolated lateral compartment osteoarthritis.

Lateral OWDFO is indicated in valgus knees with lateral meniscal deficiency, as an isolated procedure or combined with lateral meniscal transplant. Lateral meniscal transplant is generally associated in young patients (<45 years of age) with very initial stages of lateral osteoarthritis.

DFO is also commonly indicated in case of lateral compartment chondral/osteo-chondral lesions (ie, OCD) and valgus malalignment. Correcting the malalignment before or concurrently with cartilage repair is of paramount importance in order to protect the repair and unload the affected compartment.

DFOs can also be performed in case of chronic MCL deficiency. MCL reconstruction can be performed together or after realignment.[4] In some cases, mostly in older patients with low demands, DFO alone is enough to reduce MCL instability and no additional medial compartment reconstruction is needed.

In 2014, Hetsroni and colleagues[5] performed a cadaveric study to evaluate the effect of DFO on medial knee opening. They compared medial opening in 8 cadaveric specimens, with MCL and anterior cruciate ligament sectioned, before and after a lateral opening wedge DFO. They found a decrease of medial laxity at 30° of flexion after DFO in superficial MCL-transected knees.

Contraindications of OWDFO include (1) chronic inflammatory diseases, (2) severe osteoarthritis (Ahlback >III) of the lateral compartment, (3) obesity, (4) impaired range of movement, (5) osteoarthritis involving the medial and lateral compartments, (6) osteonecrosis, and (7) large corrections (>15 mm of lateral opening).[1]

PREOPERATIVE PLANNING

- A complete radiographic examination is needed to accurately plan the osteotomy, including weight-bearing anteroposterior (AP) and lateral views, skyline, Rosenberg views, and weight-bearing long leg radiographs.
- The valgus mechanical axis of the affected limb is checked by drawing the weight-bearing line from the center of the femoral head to the center of the ankle joint on the AP view of the long leg radiograph.

- Correction to a neutral alignment (no overcorrection) is planned for varus-producing osteotomies. A point located at 50% of the tibial width (between the medial and lateral tibial eminence) is marked on the AP view of the long leg radiograph (**Fig. 1**).
- Two lines are drawn connecting this point with the center of the femoral head and the center of the ankle joint.
- The acute angle (not the obtuse complementary angle) connecting these 2 lines is the angle of correction.
- Then the osteotomy line is drawn: this should be oriented from lateral to medial (ending close to the adductor tubercle) and proximal to distal (20° angle with the axis perpendicular to the femoral shaft).

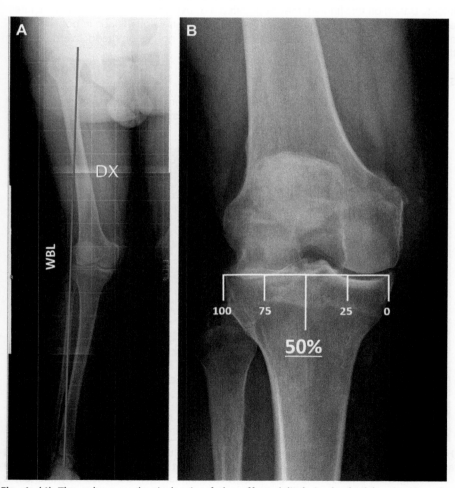

Fig. 1. (*A*) The valgus mechanical axis of the affected limb is checked by drawing the weight-bearing line (WBL) from the center of the femoral head to the center of the ankle joint on the AP view of the long leg radiograph. (*B*) Correction to a neutral alignment (no overcorrection) is planned for varus-producing osteotomies. A point located at 50% of the tibial width (between the medial and lateral tibial eminence) is marked on the AP view of the long leg radiograph.

- The length of the osteotomy is measured, and this distance transferred on both rays of the angle of correction starting from the apex.
- The base of the isosceles triangle obtained in this fashion is the opening required at the osteotomy site and the size of the spacer, when using a spacer plate (**Fig. 2**).

Although most investigators recommend a correction to neutral alignment for DFO, Quirno and colleagues[6] in their biomechanical study suggested an overcorrection of 5°. In 5 human cadaveric knees, they gradually increased the DFO angles, shifting the loading vector medially. In this way, the contact area and the contact pressure on the lateral compartment decreased, with an increase in the medial compartment. The larger reduction of contact pressure was seen at 15° of correction in 10° valgus knees. Based on this finding, they suggested a 5° overcorrection. Despite these interesting in vitro findings, we think that overcorrection in valgus knees in not well tolerated by patients in the clinical setting and we do not recommend overcorrecting these knees.

SURGICAL TECHNIQUE

- The patient is positioned supine on a radiolucent table under general or spinal anesthesia. Intravenous antibiotics are administered (usually cefazolin 2 g). A tourniquet is placed around the thigh.

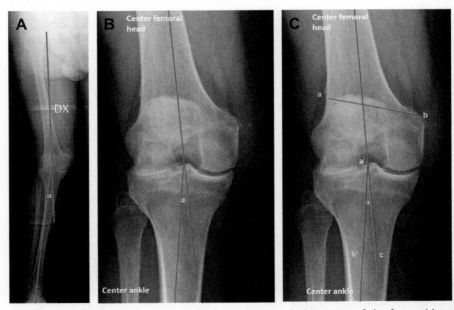

Fig. 2. (*A*) Two lines are drawn connecting this point with the center of the femoral head and the center of the ankle joint. (*B*) The acute angle (not the obtuse complementary angle) connecting these 2 lines is the angle of correction alpha. Then the osteotomy line (ab) is drawn: this should be oriented from lateral to medial (ending close to the adductor tubercle) and proximal to distal (20° angle with the axis perpendicular to the femoral shaft). (*C*) The length of the osteotomy is measured, and this distance transferred on both rays of the angle of correction starting from the apex ($a^i b^i$ and $a^i c$). The base of the isosceles triangle ($b^i c$) obtained in this fashion is the opening required at the osteotomy site and the size of the spacer, when using a spacer plate.

- Arthroscopy is performed with standard anteromedial and anterolateral portals to confirm the lateral compartment arthritis/overload, rule out medial or patellofemoral significant degeneration, and for additional procedures on the cartilage or menisci, if required.
- A 12-cm lateral femoral incision is made, starting from the lateral epicondyle and extended proximally (**Fig. 3**A). The iliotibial band is split and the vastus lateralis elevated anteriorly from the intermuscular septum (**Fig. 3**B). The lateral femoral cortex is exposed.
- Under fluoroscopic guidance, a guide wire is placed in the center of the femoral shaft from 33 fingers above the lateral epicondyle (6–7 cm above the joint line) to few millimeters proximal to the medial epicondyle (4–5 cm above the joint line) with an inclination of approximately 20° (**Fig. 4**).
- A mark on the cortex above and below the osteotomy helps to reduce the risk of rotation of the femoral fragment once the osteotomy is completed. The knee is flexed to slacken the neurovascular structures posteriorly and minimize injuries.[7]
- An oscillating saw is used to start the osteotomy proximal to the guide wire, to prevent distal migration of the osteotomy (**Fig. 5**A). The blade should be on a plane perpendicular to the coronal plane; if the cut is performed with a slope, this will result in a difficult plating (when using a spacer plate), with the proximal holes of the plate being to anterior or too posterior (according to the slope given to the osteotomy cut).
- The cut is completed with thin osteotomes to within 1 cm from the medial cortex (**Fig. 5**B). The mobility of the osteotomy is checked with gentle varus forces, to ensure the cortex has been cut anteriorly and posteriorly.
- The osteotomy is opened gradually with a wedge opener until the desired correction is obtained (**Fig. 6**A). This needs to be done gently and gradually. Compared with medial opening wedge tibial osteotomies, the medial hinge in DFO is more fragile and more prone to disruption. Medial hinge disruption may result in difficulties in controlling rotational and medial to lateral displacement of the femoral fragments.
- To assess the alignment correction with fluoroscopy, a long alignment rod is placed from the center of the femoral head to the center of the ankle (**Fig. 6**B). For a neutral alignment, the rod should pass through the center of the knee.
- Then the osteotomy can be fixed. The authors' favorite fixation device is the femoral Puddu plate (Arthrex, Naples, FL) (**Fig. 7**). This is a titanium T-shaped tooth plate with 3 distal holes for cancellous screws and 4 proximal holes for bicortical screws.[8] Alternatively, a locking lateral plate without spacer (ie, TomoFix plate; Depuy Synthes, Raynham, MA) can be used. Both plating devices provide adequate fixation strength, and this is generally a matter of preference of the

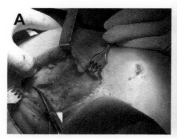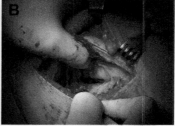

Fig. 3. Surgical technique (see text). (*A*) Lateral incision. (*B*) Elevation of the vastus lateralis muscle.

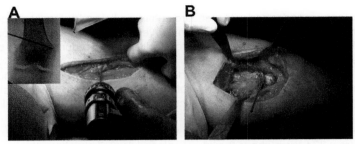

Fig. 4. Surgical technique (see text). (*A*) Insertion of the guide wire under fluoroscopic guidance (panel). (*B*) Guide wire in place and osteotomy line drawn with the electrocautery.

    surgeon. Both devices require hardware removal in a significant percentage of patients, because of irritation of the iliotibial band.[9]

- After plating is performed, the osteotomy gap is generally bone grafted. Different options are available, including iliac crest autograft, allograft, and bone substitutes. The authors' favorite bone grafting option is femoral head allograft. Two wedges are obtained from the femoral head and used to fill the osteotomy gap.
- Postoperatively, the patient is kept in a hinged knee brace for 6 weeks with free range of motion and toe touch weight-bearing. The patient is generally progressed to weight bearing as tolerated at 6 to 8 weeks from surgery (depending on the amount of correction and radiographic healing of the osteotomy).

DISCUSSION

DFO for lateral osteoarthritis is a less common procedure compared with high tibial osteotomy for the varus knee, probably because of the lower incidence of genu valgum. As a consequence, the literature about this topic is sparse.

In a recent review, Kim and colleagues[10] reported nonsignificant differences in clinical and radiological outcomes between opening wedge and closing wedge DFO, with the closing wedge technique being more technically demanding.

Opening wedge DFO has shown good results with a low rate of conversion to arthroplasty.

Saithna and colleagues[11] reported a cumulative survival rate of DFOs of 79% at 5 years, Madelaine and colleagues[12] reported an even higher survival rate of 91.4% at 5 years.

Chahla and colleagues,[13] in a systematic review of 14 studies (9 studies regarding CWDFO and 5 OWDFO), reported a survival rate between 82% and 100% at 6 to 8 years for OWDFO.

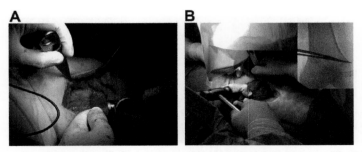

Fig. 5. Surgical technique (see text). (*A*) The osteotomy is started with an oscillating saw. (*B*) The osteotomy is completed with osteotomes under fluoroscopic guidance (panel).

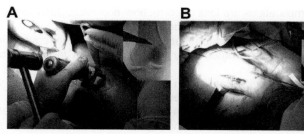

Fig. 6. Surgical technique (see text). (*A*) The osteotomy is then opened with graduated wedges under fluoroscopic guidance (panel). (*B*) The alignment is then checked with a long alignment rod and the fluoroscope.

Wylie and colleagues[14] reviewed 7 studies (137 osteotomies) and reported that the conversion to total knee arthroplasty (TKA) was 12% at 45 to 78 months of mean follow-up.

In a recent study by Elattar and colleagues[15] on 28 patients (41 DFOs) with a mean follow-up of 26 months (range 12–57), no patients required a total knee replacement.

Cameron and colleagues[16] demonstrated a higher survival rate in patients who required a DFO associated with a cartilage repair or meniscal transplantation. They stratified the patients into 2 groups: osteoarthritis group (19 knees) and joint preservation group (12 knees); this last group included patients who underwent osteochondral allograft transplantation or meniscal allograft transplantation. Conversion to TKA at 5 years was lower in the joint preservation group. Mean International Knee Documentation Committee score improved from 47 to 67 after the surgery for the arthritis group, and from 36 to 62 for the joint preservation group.

Complications associated with DFO can be divided into intraoperative and postoperative.

The most common intraoperative complications are intra-articular fractures and breaches of the medial hinge. An incomplete osteotomy or a guide pin placed too close to the joint can cause an intra-articular fracture.[1,7]

Other possible complications include neurovascular injuries. Van der Woude and colleagues[17] performed a cadaveric study about periosteal vascularization of distal femur. They suggested using the lateral transverse artery as a landmark for finding the height of the osteotomy. Transection of this artery does not result in vascular damage because of the many anastomoses in the periosteal vascularization of the lateral condyle.

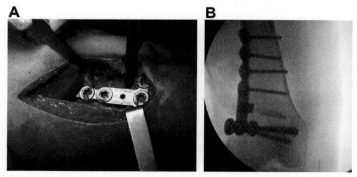

Fig. 7. Surgical technique (see text). (*A*) Plating can then be performed. (*B*) Final AP fluoroscopic view after plating and bone grafting with bone substitutes.

Postoperative complications are loss of correction, nonunion, deep venous thrombosis, compartment syndrome, and infections.

The risk of nonunion is calculated to be approximately 5%.[7] Inadequate fixation or too aggressive rehabilitation protocols may result in implant failure or osteotomy collapse with loss of correction.

For DFOs, no fixation device has shown superiority over the others. In vitro, the TomoFix plate seems to provide a greater torsional and axial stability compared with the Puddu plate, but this has not been confirmed in clinical trials.[18] Batista and colleagues[19] compared locking plate and angle blade plate constructs on 48 synthetic femora after a lateral opening wedge DFO. The investigators performed axial and torsional tests on 2 groups: one with intact medial cortex and one with fractured medial cortex. In the fractured group they also evaluated the effect of a 6.5-mm cancellous screw placed on the medial cortex. They concluded that angle blade plate provided more stiffness for torsional loads and axial compression. In addition, the medial screw placed on a fractured medial hinge provided stability similar to an intact medial cortex. Recently, Kim and colleagues,[10] in a systematic review comparing opening and closing wedge DFOs, found that the Puddu plate is comparable to the angle blade plate and the TomoFix plate.

Hardware removal is very common in DFO. Jacobi and colleagues[9] reported 86% of plate removal after an OWDFO, due to friction on the ileo-tibial band.

To fill the osteotomy gap, bone grafts or bone substitutes can be used, including autograft, allograft, or synthetic graft (ie, calcium phosphate cement). Although the gold standard is still iliac crest autograft, the harvest entails increased surgical time and donor site morbidity. For this reason, allografts and bone substitute are commonly used with good results, and sometimes in association with platelet-rich plasma and bone marrow stromal cells.[20] Dewilde and colleagues[21] used a calcium phosphate bone cement graft in opening wedge DFO fixed with the Puddu plate and reported no delayed union. However, no conclusion can be drawn on the optimal graft choice, because of the variability of the grafts used in the studies about opening wedge DFO.[10]

SUMMARY

In conclusion, DFO is an effective treatment for young and active patients with genu valgum and lateral compartment osteoarthritis. Careful patient selection and accurate surgical technique are fundamental in achieving good results. Closing and opening wedge techniques show similar results. OWDFO is technically easier but requires bone or synthetic grafting to fill the osteotomy gap and has a higher risk of delayed union.

REFERENCES

1. Rosso F, Margheritini F. Distal femoral osteotomy. Curr Rev Musculoskelet Med 2014;7:302–11.

2. Thienpont E, Schwab PE, Cornu O, et al. Bone morphotypes of the varus and valgus knee. Arch Orthop Trauma Surg 2017;137(3):393–400.

3. Eberbach H, Mehl J, Feucht MJ, et al. Geometry of the valgus knee: contradicting the dogma of a femoral-based deformity. Am J Sports Med 2017;45(4):909–14.

4. Phisitkul P, Wolf BR, Amendola A. Role of high tibial and distal femoral osteotomies in the treatment of lateral-posterolateral and medial instabilities of the knee. Sports Med Arthrosc Rev 2006;14(2):96–104.

5. Hetsroni I, Lyman S, Pearle AD, et al. The effect of lateral opening wedge distal femoral osteotomy on medial knee opening: clinical and biomechanical factors. Knee Surg Sports Traumatol Arthrosc 2014;22(7):1659–65.
6. Quirno M, Campbell KA, Singh B, et al. Distal femoral varus osteotomy for unloading valgus knee malalignment: a biomechanical analysis. Knee Surg Sports Traumatol Arthrosc 2017;25(3):863–8.
7. O'Malley MP, Pareek A, Reardon PJ, et al. Distal femoral osteotomy: lateral opening wedge technique. Arthrosc Tech 2016;5(4):e725–30.
8. Puddu GCM, Cerullo G, Franco V, et al. Which osteotomy for a valgus knee? Int Orthop 2010;34(2):239–47. The original technique about opening wedge DFO performed with the Puddu Plate®.].
9. Jacobi M, Wahl P, Bouaicha S, et al. Distal femoral varus osteotomy: problems associated with the lateral open-wedge technique. Arch Orthop Trauma Surg 2011;131(6):725–8.
10. Kim YC, Yang JH, Kim HJ, et al. Distal femoral varus osteotomy for valgus arthritis of the knees: systematic review of open versus closed wedge osteotomy. Knee Surg Relat Res 2018;30(1):3–16.
11. Saithna A, Kundra R, Getgood A, et al. Opening wedge distal femoral varus osteotomy for lateral compartment osteoarthritis in the valgus knee. Knee 2014;21: 172–5.
12. Madelaine A, Lording T, Villa V, et al. The effect of lateral opening wedge distal femoral osteotomy on leg length. Knee Surg Sports Traumatol Arthrosc 2016; 24:847–54.
13. Chahla J, Mitchell JJ, Liechti DJ, et al. Opening- and closing-wedge distal femoral osteotomy: a systematic review of outcomes for isolated lateral compartment osteoarthritis. Orthop J Sports Med 2016;4. 2325967116649901.
14. Wylie JD, Jones DL, Hartley MK, et al. Distal femoral osteotomy for the valgus knee: medial closing wedge versus lateral opening wedge: a systematic review. Arthroscopy 2016;32(10):2141–7.
15. Elattar O, Swarup I, Lam A, et al. Open wedge distal femoral osteotomy: accuracy of correction and patient outcomes. HSS J 2017;13(2):128–35.
16. Cameron JI, McCauley JC, Kermanshahi AY, et al. Lateral opening-wedge distal femoral osteotomy: pain relief, functional improvement, and survivorship at 5 years. Clin Orthop Relat Res 2015;473(6):2009–15.
17. van der Woude JA, van Heerwaarden RJ, Bleys RL. Periosteal vascularization of the distal femur in relation to distal femoral osteotomies: a cadaveric study. J Exp Orthop 2016;3(1):6.
18. Stoffel K, Stachowiak G, Kuster M. Open wedge high tibial osteotomy: biomechanical investigation of the modified arthrex osteotomy plate (Puddu Plate) and the TomoFix plate. Clin Biomech (Bristol, Avon) 2004;19(9):944–50.
19. Batista BB, Volpon JB, Shimano AC, et al. Varization open-wedge osteotomy of the distal femur: comparison between locking plate and angle blade plate constructs. Knee Surg Sports Traumatol Arthrosc 2015;23(8):2202–7.
20. Dallari D, Savarino L, Stagni C, et al. Enhanced tibial osteotomy healing with use of bone grafts supplemented with platelet gel or platelet gel and bone marrow stromal cells. J Bone Joint Surg Am 2007;89(11):2413–20.
21. Dewilde TR, Dauw J, Vandenneucker H, et al. Opening wedge distal femoral varus osteotomy using the puddu plate and calcium phosphate bone cement. Knee Surg Sports Traumatol Arthrosc 2013;21:249–54.

Medial Closing Wedge Distal Femoral Osteotomy

Nicholas C. Duethman, MD[a,b], Christopher D. Bernard, BS[a,b],
Christopher L. Camp, MD[a,b], Aaron J. Krych, MD[a,b], Michael J. Stuart, MD[a,b],*

KEYWORDS

- Genu valgus • Distal medial femoral osteotomy • Lateral compartment arthritis

KEY POINTS

- Valgus malalignment of the knee joint is present when the mechanical axis of the lower extremity is lateral to the center of the knee.
- Medial shift of the mechanical axis can be accomplished by a medial distal femoral closing wedge osteotomy.
- Poor preoperative planning or surgical undercorrection/overcorrection results in improper mechanical axis alignment.
- The ideal candidates are young and active individuals with isolated lateral compartment arthritis.

INTRODUCTION

Valgus malalignment of the knee joint is present when the mechanical axis of the lower extremity is lateral to the center of the knee. This malalignment in the coronal plane leads to increased contact stresses in the lateral compartment and can translate into early-onset degenerative joint disease.[1,2] Osteotomies around the knee can help correct alignment and serve as joint-sparing operations depending on the underlying cause of the deformity. These techniques are most often indicated in young and active individuals with unicompartmental disease.

A varus-producing osteotomy is a joint preservation technique that produces a neutral mechanical axis through the knee center. The mechanical axis is shifted medially by either a medial distal femoral or proximal tibial closing wedge osteotomy. Alternatively, it can be accomplished using a lateral distal femoral or

Investigation performed at the Mayo Clinic, Rochester, MN.
Disclosure: The authors report no actual or potential conflict of interest in relation to this article.
[a] Department of Orthopedic Surgery, Mayo Clinic, 200 First Street South West, Rochester, MN 55905, USA; [b] Department of Sports Medicine, Mayo Clinic, 200 First Street South West, Rochester, MN 55905, USA
* Corresponding author.
E-mail address: Stuart.michael@mayo.edu

Clin Sports Med 38 (2019) 361–373
https://doi.org/10.1016/j.csm.2019.02.005
0278-5919/19/© 2019 Elsevier Inc. All rights reserved.

sportsmed.theclinics.com

proximal tibial opening wedge osteotomy. The site of the osteotomy is dictated by the location of the deformity. A lateral opening wedge and medial closing wedge both have advantages and disadvantages. The focus of this article is the medial distal femoral closing wedge osteotomy to correct valgus malalignment in the setting of lateral compartment arthritis or recurrent lateral patellar instability.

INDICATIONS

In order to determine the degree of malalignment as well as the level of deformity, high-quality full-length, standing, hip-to-ankle radiographs are required. The technique should ensure that there is no malrotation and full knee extension. The anatomic and mechanical axes as well as the weight-bearing line of the lower extremity are measured. If the mechanical axis passes lateral to the center of the knee, this defines a valgus deformity (**Fig. 1**). To determine the level of deformity (femoral vs tibial), measure the lateral distal femoral angle created by the mechanical axis of the femur and a line drawn transversely across the articular surface of the femoral condyles (**Fig. 2**). The typical value is between 85° and 90°.[3] A value lower than this represents a hypoplastic lateral femoral condyle, implicating the femur as the location of the deformity. If this measurement is within normal limits, evaluate the tibia by determining the medial proximal tibial angle created by a line through the mechanical axis of the tibia and a horizontal line across the medial and lateral tibial plateaus (**Fig. 3**). Normal values are between 85° and 90°.[3] Larger values implicate the tibia as the site of the deformity.

Tibial malalignment is a contraindication to a distal femoral osteotomy (DFO). Osteochondral lesions and meniscus deficiency can lead to a valgus deformity and should be addressed before the osteotomy in order to ensure proper angular correction. Similarly, a valgus deformity could be caused by soft tissue laxity on the medial side of the knee, and soft tissue procedures could be indicated rather than osteotomy. Advanced arthritis and multicompartment involvement are contraindications to DFO and are best treated with knee arthroplasty. Indications and contraindications are summarized in **Table 1**.

PREOPERATIVE PLANNING
Radiographic Templating

Obtain a full series of radiographs, including standing anteroposterior (AP), lateral, patellar, and posteroanterior flexion views of the knee, along with a full-length standing view of the lower extremity. MRI is indicated if meniscal or osteochondral defects are suspected.

Using a high-quality hip-to-ankle standing film, draw the weight-bearing line from the center of the femoral head to the center of the talus. A valgus deformity is present if this line passes lateral to the center of the knee. The angle of the osteotomy is determined based on a neutral (0°) mechanical axis of the limb (**Fig. 4**). This angle is formed by lines drawn from the center of the femoral head and the center of the talus to the center of the knee (**Fig. 5**). Five degrees is the smallest practical angle amenable to an osteotomy. The measured correction angle can be drawn onto a calibrated AP radiograph of the knee at the planned osteotomy site. The size of the wedge is measured as the distance between the proximal and distal cuts on the medial femoral cortex. The location of the supracondylar osteotomy is determined by the position of the precontoured plate, as discussed later.

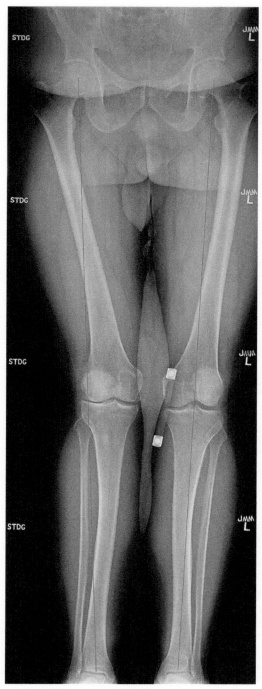

Fig. 1. Full-length standing radiograph showing valgus deformity of the right knee with the weight-bearing line passing through the periphery of the lateral compartment.

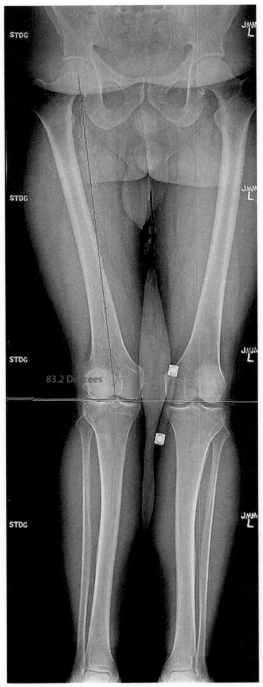

Fig. 2. Determining the level of deformity (femoral vs tibial): The lateral distal femoral angle is measured as an angle created by the mechanical axis of the femur and a line drawn transversely across the articular surface of the lateral femoral condyles.

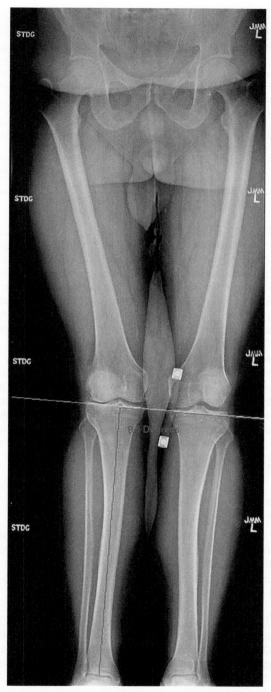

Fig. 3. Measurement of the medial proximal tibial angle by drawing a line through the mechanical axis of the tibia and a horizontal line across the medial and lateral tibial plateaus.

| Table 1 |
| Indications and contraindications of distal femoral varus osteotomy |

Indications:	Relative contraindications:
• Valgus knee malalignment >5°	• Symptomatic or moderate to severe patellofemoral osteoarthritis
• Isolated lateral compartment mild to moderate osteoarthritis	• High body mass index
• Lateral condyle cartilage lesions	• Nicotine use
• Deficiency of meniscus in the lateral compartment	• Age >55 y
• Desire to remain active	Absolute contraindications:
• Young and middle-aged patients (<55 y old)	• Severe medial or tricompartmental osteoarthritis
	• Inflammatory arthritis
	• Severe osteoporosis
	• Knee flexion <90°

Technique Selection

The distal femur is the preferred site for surgical correction of valgus malalignment because a hypoplastic lateral femoral condyle is often associated with this deformity.[4,5] A medial closing wedge or a lateral opening wedge DFO may be performed. There is no clear evidence that one technique is superior to the other. The advantages of performing a medial closing wedge osteotomy are direct bone apposition, construct stability, reliable bone healing, no need for bone graft, inherent stability allowing immediate partial weight bearing, and medial access for concomitant procedures through a single incision.[6,7] The disadvantages include decreased familiarity with the surgical exposure for some clinicians, increased risk for neurovascular injury caused by proximity to the popliteal vessels, and less ability to fine-tune the intraoperative correction.[6,8] The advantages of performing a lateral opening wedge osteotomy are a familiar surgical approach, single bone cut, better control of the intraoperative correction, and access to the lateral aspect of the knee where the disorder is most commonly found enabling concomitant procedures.[4,5,7] The disadvantages include a need for bone graft, longer time to bony healing, increased risk of malunion or nonunion, potential hardware irritation, and non–weight-bearing ambulation for 8 weeks postoperatively.[4,5,9]

SURGICAL TECHNIQUE
Operative Preparation

General or spinal anesthesia is induced with an optional peripheral nerve block for postoperative pain control. The patient is placed in a supine position on a standard operating table. Before draping, sample fluoroscopic images are taken to ensure optimal patient position for required radiographs. The operative limb may be elevated to facilitate lateral radiographs.

Surgical Approach

A medial longitudinal skin incision is centered over the epicondyle, approximately 10 cm in length. Dissection is carried down to the fascial layer overlying the vastus medialis and stopped proximal to the knee joint. The vastus medialis is then elevated anteriorly with electrocautery or scissors along the anterior margin of the intermuscular septum (**Fig. 6**A). Care is taken to cauterize all perforating vessels. Visualization is optimized with 2 Bennett retractors on the anterior femoral cortex, reflecting the vastus medialis anteriorly (**Fig. 6**B).

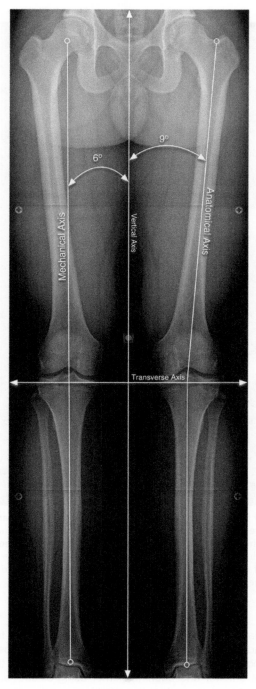

Fig. 4. The normal mechanical and anatomic axes of the lower limb in a bilateral standing full-length anteroposterior radiograph. The mechanical axis follows a line from the femoral head through the center of the talus. The anatomic axis follows a line through the center of the femoral shaft through the center of the tibia to the center of the ankle.[4]

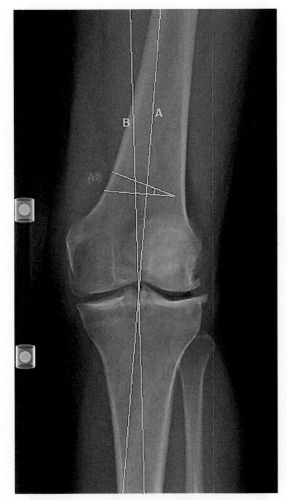

Fig. 5. Calculation of the correction angle to create a neutral (0°) mechanical axis. This cropped view at the knee shows how the deformity correction is determined. The line A runs from the center of the femoral head passing through the center of the knee. B runs from the center of the talus to the center of the knee. The resultant angle of lines A and B is the desired angle of correction. Angle AB represents the location and orientation of the medial closing wedge osteotomy.[6]

Osteotomy

A precontoured plate is placed on the medial femur external to the periosteum (**Fig. 6**C). The metadiaphyseal region is marked at the site of the osteotomy between the plate screw holes. A transverse medial incision through the periosteum is extended along the anterior and posterior femur using electrocautery. A malleable retractor is placed anteriorly to protect the quadriceps and posteriorly to protect the neurovascular structures.

The osteotomy is outlined by placing 2 bicortical Kirschner wires from medial to lateral corresponding with the planned osteotomy angle and the cortical length of

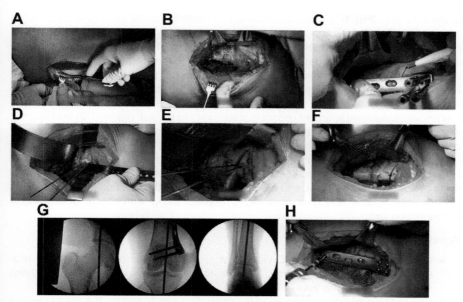

Fig. 6. (*A*) Exposure for planned osteotomy site: The vastus medialis muscle is elevated ante-riorly using scissors, staying along the anterior margin of the intermuscular septum. (*B*) Two Bennett retractors are placed on the anterior femoral cortex with reflexion of the vastus me-dialis anteriorly to optimize visualization. (*C*) Planning of the osteotomy site: a precon-toured locking distal femoral plate is placed on the distal medial femur external to the periosteum. The osteotomy site is marked at the metaphyseal-diaphyseal region proximal to the distal locking screws using electrocautery. (*D*) Two bicortical Kirschner wires are placed medial to lateral at the angle of the planned osteotomy using the previously described geometric triangular method. (*E*) The wedge osteotomy is created using an oscil-lating saw between the 2 Kirschner wires, preserving approximately 5 mm of lateral cortex. (*F*) The osteotomy is closed using a gentle, steady, varus-directed force on the lower leg while stabilizing the knee. (*G*) Final mechanical axis views are obtained for confirmation of accurate alignment. The mechanical axis as shown proceeds from the center of the femoral head through the center of the knee joint and to the center of the talus. (*H*) Once alignment has been confirmed, the remaining distal locking holes are filled with screws.

triangle base (**Fig. 6**D). A longitudinal mark is placed on the medial cortex of the femur using electrocautery as a perpendicular referencing guide to avoid malrotation. The wedge osteotomy is created using an oscillating saw between the 2 Kirschner wires preserving approximately 5 mm of lateral femoral cortex (**Fig. 6**E). Copious irrigation is used to avoid thermal injury from the saw. The wedge of bone is then removed. Additional cortical release is sometimes necessary on the anterior and posterior femur using a small osteotome (**Fig. 6**H). The 2 Kirschner wires are then removed. The osteotomy is closed using a gentle varus-directed force on the lower leg while stabi-lizing the knee (**Fig. 6**F).

The precontoured medial distal femoral locking plate is placed and pinned proxi-mally and distally with the solid portion of the plate over the osteotomy site. A self-tapping, locking screw is inserted distally through the plate. Alignment is confirmed using AP fluoroscopy and a long metal rod to verify that the weight-bearing line from the center of the femoral head to the center of the talus passes through the center of the knee joint (**Fig. 6**G). Once confirmed, the remaining distal locking holes are filled with screws (**Fig. 6**H). Compression across the osteotomy site is then achieved by using a cortical screw placed through the first hole proximal to the osteotomy. The screw is directed in a proximal to lateral trajectory in order to maximize compression across this osteotomy site. The remaining 3 holes are filled using unicortical locking screws. Plate position is then verified with AP and lateral fluoroscopy.

The timing of concomitant procedures, such as an osteochondral lesion repair or a medial patellofemoral ligament reconstruction, should be well planned. In scenarios in which deep flexion will be required, it is better to perform this procedure before the osteotomy to avoid flexing the femur with new hardware in place.

Hemostasis is obtained and the wound is thoroughly irrigated. The vastus medialis is reattached to the intermuscular septum with absorbable suture, subcutaneous tissue closed with 2-0 Monocryl, and the skin closed with 3-0 subcuticular running stitch. An occlusive gauze and glue dressing is applied along with sterile gauze and a compression wrap.

Pearls

- When combining medial DFO with other procedures, perform intraarticular procedures before the osteotomy. Manipulating the lower extremity after applying the plate can lead to loss of fixation.
- Use copious irrigation when using the oscillating saw to reduce the risk of thermal injury and bone necrosis.
- Preserve 5 mm of lateral cortex when making the osteotomy to serve as a hinge.
- Close the osteotomy gap slowly by carefully applying continuous manual compression to the lateral lower limb in a varus direction while stabilizing the knee joint to avoid fracture of the lateral cortex.

Pitfalls

- Poor preoperative planning, overcorrection, or undercorrection can lead to improper mechanical axis alignment.
- If malleable retractors are not properly placed both anteriorly and posteriorly, iatrogenic injury to either the quadriceps or neurovascular structures may occur.
- Fracture of the lateral cortex at the site of the osteotomy may decrease stability.

POSTOPERATIVE REGIMEN

A chemoprophylaxis agent is administered to prevent deep venous thrombosis based on the individual's preoperative risk factors.[4] For the first 6 weeks following the procedure, the patient's leg is placed in a knee brace that is locked in full extension for partial weight bearing and unlocked for knee range of motion to a maximum of 90°.[6,10] After 6 weeks, the brace is discontinued, crutches are weaned, and the patient may begin quadriceps strengthening and full range of motion. The patient should not load the knee at flexion angles greater than 90°. At 3 months postoperative, knee radiographs, including a full-length standing hip-to-ankle radiograph view, are obtained to assess bone healing and alignment correction. A gradual return to activity and sport-specific training can occur in a progressive fashion as tolerated by the patient.[4,6,10]

RESULTS

There is consistency in the orthopedic literature with regard to patient outcomes and longevity following a medial closing wedge DFO operation. Positive survival rates, indicating that patients have not converted to a total knee arthroplasty, can be appreciated in the short term with an increased failure rate after 10 years postoperatively. In 41 patients who underwent 45 DFO procedures, Sternheim and colleagues[11] showed a survival rate of 89.9% at 10 years postoperatively, 78.9% at 15 years, and 21.5% at 20 years. The same study showed improvement in mean modified Knee Society scores from 36.1 preoperatively to 74.4 at 1 year postoperatively, and 60.5 at latest follow-up. Patients who underwent bilateral DFO and those with a higher body mass index had worse outcomes. Backstein and colleagues[12] reported on 40 DFO procedures with a 10-year survival rate of 82%, but a 15-year survival rate of only 45%. At the most recent follow-up, 60% reported good or excellent results, whereas 15% had fair or poor results, with most of the latter group awaiting total knee arthroplasty.

In a systematic review, Chahla and colleagues[13] showed that survivorship rates after medial closing wedge DFO were initially strong, with progressive decline over time. Survival rates varied from 83%[14] to 92%[15] at 4 years' follow-up, 64%[16] to 89.9%[11] at 10 years' follow-up, and 45%[12] to 78.9%[11] at 15 years' follow-up. One study showed survival of 21.5%[11] at 20 years after surgery. All studies that provided patient-reported outcome scores showed improvement from the osteotomy.[13] A systematic review by Wylie and colleagues[17] reported a survival rate of 100% at a mean of 5 years and 52% at a mean of 15 years postoperatively. In the same review, a variety of patient-reported outcome scores were used, with mean improvement in those scores postoperatively.

Complications

There are vast discrepancies regarding the complication rate with DFO in the literature, ranging from 0% to 63%.[17–20] Intraarticular fracture can occur if the guide pin is positioned too close to the joint or if the osteotomy is not extended far enough laterally.[21] In a study performed by Edgerton and colleagues,[20] 25% of patients developed a nonunion and 21% lost correction. Mathews and colleagues[19] reported on their cohort of 21 patients, showing that 57% experienced a significant complication, including 48% with severe knee stiffness requiring manipulation under anesthesia, 19% with nonunion or delayed union, 10% with an infection, and 5% with fixation failure. These rates seem to be decreasing with improved techniques, because the risk of osteotomy nonunion is reported as 5% of cases in the literature, with delayed union taking up to 6 months in some circumstances.[4] Although it is presumed that there is less symptomatic hardware in a medial closing wedge osteotomy compared with a lateral opening wedge osteotomy because of friction between the plate and iliotibial band, the reported rates are similar.[13,17] The most devastating complication of DFO is injury to the popliteal neurovascular bundle.[5] This injury may occur with either unintentional perforation of the posterior femoral cortex or poor retractor placement. Kim and colleagues[22] analyzed the distance between the popliteal artery and the posterior cortex of the tibia in fresh-frozen cadaveric lower extremities at various degrees of knee flexion and found that neurovascular structures are furthest from the tibia when the knee is in 90° of flexion.

SUMMARY

The orthopedic literature contains fewer reports on the results of DFO compared with proximal tibial osteotomy because valgus malalignment is less common. Ideal candidates for distal femoral varus-producing osteotomy are young and active individuals with isolated lateral compartment arthritis and valgus malalignment. The goal of the procedure is to create a neutral mechanical axis of the limb to relieve pain and preserve the knee joint. The amount of correction is calculated from a preoperative, high-quality, weight-bearing radiograph from the hip to ankle. This technically challenging operation is a viable option for patients with valgus malalignment because early survivorship is strong and patient-reported outcome scores are significantly improved.

ACKNOWLEDGMENTS

O'Malley et al: **Fig. 4**. Sabbag et al: **Fig. 5**.

REFERENCES

1. Sharma L, Song J, Felson D, et al. The role of knee alignment in disease progression and functional decline in knee osteoarthritis. JAMA 2001;286(2):188–95.
2. Tetsworth K, Paley D. Malalignment and degenerative arthropathy. Orthop Clin North Am 1994;25(3):367–77.
3. Paley D, Herzenberg JE, Tetsworth K, et al. Deformity planning for frontal and sagittal plane corrective osteotomies. Orthop Clin North Am 1994;25(3):425–65.
4. O'Malley MP, Pareek A, Reardon PJ, et al. Distal femoral osteotomy: lateral opening wedge technique. Arthrosc Tech 2016;5(4):e725–30.
5. Olivero M, Rosso F, Dettoni F, et al. Femoral osteotomies for the valgus knee. Ann Joint 2017;2(6):4–12.
6. Sabbag OD, Woodmass JM, Wu IT, et al. Medial closing-wedge distal femoral osteotomy with medial patellofemoral ligament imbrication for genu valgum with lateral patellar instability. Arthrosc Tech 2017;6(6):e2085–91.
7. Wylie JD, Maak TG. Medial closing-wedge distal femoral osteotomy for genu valgum with lateral compartment disease. Arthrosc Tech 2016;5(6):e1357–66.
8. Tirico LE, Demange MK, Bonadio MB, et al. Medial closing-wedge distal femoral osteotomy: fixation with proximal tibial locking plate. Arthrosc Tech 2015;4(6):e687–95.
9. Mitchell JJ, Dean CS, Chahla J, et al. Varus-producing lateral distal femoral opening-wedge osteotomy. Arthrosc Tech 2016;5(4):e799–807.
10. Voleti PB, Wu IT, Degen RM, et al. Successful return to sport following distal femoral varus osteotomy. Cartilage 2017;10(1):19–25.
11. Sternheim A, Garbedian S, Backstein D. Distal femoral varus osteotomy: unloading the lateral compartment: long-term follow-up of 45 medial closing wedge osteotomies. Orthopedics 2011;34(9):e488–90.
12. Backstein D, Morag G, Hanna S, et al. Long-term follow-up of distal femoral varus osteotomy of the knee. J Arthroplasty 2007;22(4 Suppl 1):2–6.
13. Chahla J, Mitchell JJ, Liechti DJ, et al. Opening- and closing-wedge distal femoral osteotomy: a systematic review of outcomes for isolated lateral compartment osteoarthritis. Orthop J Sports Med 2016;4(6). 2325967116649901.
14. Healy WL, Anglen JO, Wasilewski SA, et al. Distal femoral varus osteotomy. J Bone Joint Surg Am 1988;70(1):102–9.
15. McDermott AG, Finklestein JA, Farine I, et al. Distal femoral varus osteotomy for valgus deformity of the knee. J Bone Joint Surg Am 1988;70(1):110–6.
16. Finkelstein JA, Gross AE, Davis A. Varus osteotomy of the distal part of the femur. A survivorship analysis. J Bone Joint Surg Am 1996;78(9):1348–52.
17. Wylie JD, Jones DL, Hartley MK, et al. Distal femoral osteotomy for the valgus knee: medial closing wedge versus lateral opening wedge: a systematic review. Arthroscopy 2016;32(10):2141–7.

18. Learmonth ID. A simple technique for varus supracondylar osteotomy in genu valgum. J Bone Joint Surg Br 1990;72(2):235–7.
19. Mathews J, Cobb AG, Richardson S, et al. Distal femoral osteotomy for lateral compartment osteoarthritis of the knee. Orthopedics 1998;21(4):437–40.
20. Edgerton BC, Mariani EM, Morrey BF. Distal femoral varus osteotomy for painful genu valgum. A five-to-11-year follow-up study. Clin Orthop Relat Res 1993;(288): 263–9.
21. Puddu G, Cipolla M, Cerullo G, et al. Osteotomies: the surgical treatment of the valgus knee. Sports Med Arthrosc Rev 2007;15(1):15–22.
22. Kim J, Allaire R, Harner CD. Vascular safety during high tibial osteotomy: a cadaveric angiographic study. Am J Sports Med 2010;38(4):810–5.

Lateral Closing Wedge High Tibial Osteotomy for Medial Compartment Arthrosis or Overload

Giulio Maria Marcheggiani Muccioli, MD, PhD[a],
Stefano Fratini, MD[b],*, Eugenio Cammisa, MD[b],
Vittorio Vaccari, MD[b], Alberto Grassi, MD[b],
Laura Bragonzoni, PhD[c], Stefano Zaffagnini, MD[b]

KEYWORDS

- Knee • Surgery • Osteotomy • Lateral closing wedge • Cartilage • Arthrosis

KEY POINTS

- Osteotomy can be a valid alternative to total knee arthroplasty in selected patients.
- The ideal candidate for a high tibial osteotomy is a young patient (<60 years of age) with isolated medial osteoarthritis (OA) and good range of motion, and without ligamentous instability.
- Lateral closing wedge osteotomies are an effective treatment of unicompartmental arthrosis or deformities.
- Correct execution of surgery is crucial, the weightbearing line should pass through the lateral 30% to 40% of the tibial plateau. Preoperative planning is mandatory to achieve this result.
- The postoperative regimen must include 6 months of partial weightbearing, then full weightbearing if radiological consolidation of the fracture is visible.

INTRODUCTION

Osteotomy is among the most ancient type of orthopedic treatment. It has been in existence for more than 2000 years[1] and it is still used currently. The basic principle is to perform a bone cut to allow realignment of the deformity-affected limb or segment.

---

[a] II Clinica Ortopedica e Traumatologica, Istituto Ortopedico Rizzoli, Lab Biomeccanica, via di Barbiano, 1/10, Bologna 40136, Italy; [b] II Clinica Ortopedica e Traumatologica, Istituto Ortopedico Rizzoli, Bologna, Italy; [c] Laboratorio di Biomeccanica e Innovazione Tecnologica, Istituto Ortopedico Rizzoli, Bologna, Italy
* Corresponding author.
E-mail address: dr.stefano.fratini@gmail.com

Clin Sports Med 38 (2019) 375–386
https://doi.org/10.1016/j.csm.2019.02.002
0278-5919/19/© 2019 Elsevier Inc. All rights reserved.

Throughout the last century, osteotomy was widely used to treat a variety of knee deformities, including rickets, poliomyelitis, tuberculosis, and posttraumatic deformity.

The history of osteotomy originated with R. Barthon (1794–1871) but it was W. Macewen[2] who fully codified the guidelines of this procedure in the 1880. V. Putti[3,4] traced the way to angular deformities correction through osteotomy in Italy. In the United Kingdom, Jackson[5] first reported high tibial osteotomy (HTO) to treat OA of the knee. This idea was refined by Coventry[6] and Insall and colleagues,[7] who increased the popularity of lateral closing wedge HTO in the United States. In the 1980s and 1990s, there was a decrease in the use of HTO due to (1) the procedure's limitations (ie, it is not the ideal treatment of multicompartmental disease; its results progressively deteriorate because of a large heterogeneous group of patients) and (2) the success of total knee arthroplasty (TKA).

However, in recent years, the relegation of the osteotomy to his historic role has been challenged by an increased interest in the procedure as an alternative to TKA and unicompartmental knee arthroplasty in younger patients with high physical demands.

Today, new knowledge and technology about bone healing and better fixations to accelerate postoperative management have allowed HTO to become a useful procedure for active patients younger than 60 years of age with symptomatic unicompartmental disease and osseous deformity. An important advantage of this procedure is the possibility of combining the articular cartilage procedure (osteochondral grafts, autologous chondrocyte implantation), meniscus transplantation, or ligament reconstruction.

The normal anatomic loadbearing axis of the knee ranges from 5° to 7° of valgus. In a normal knee, 60% of the weight is supported by the medial compartment and 40% by the lateral compartment.[8]

Medial gonarthrosis in a varus knee is an increasingly common occurrence. Varus alignment causes an increased load on the medial compartment. For varus gonarthrosis, the main osteotomy options include proximal tibial lateral closing wedge osteotomy (LCWO), proximal tibial medial opening wedge osteotomy, dome osteotomy, or combinations of the above. The goal of all these procedures is to shift the mechanical axis laterally, traditionally at 62% to 66% of the tibial width,[8] allowing a decreased load to be transmitted to the medial compartment.

The aim of this article is to focus on LCWO, remembering that surgery goals are to relieve pain; to redistribute weightbearing forces; to improve function; and, therefore, potentially increase the longevity of the native knee joint.

INDICATIONS

Selecting the right patient is crucial in achieving good results with HTO for medial knee arthrosis. Proper patient selection and a clinical assessment are necessary when considering a closing wedge osteotomy for gonarthrosis. This assessment should include a detailed history, including age, occupation, activity level, past medical and surgical history, and patient expectations, especially their expectations of postoperative activity level. Physical examination should focus on lower extremity range of motion (hip, knee, ankle, and foot), deformity, ligamentous stability, and leg length discrepancy.[9,10]

HTO should preferably performed in a young and active patient with unicompartmental knee gonarthrosis However, it should be also considered in older patients with unicompartmental arthrosis and the desire to participate in high-impact physical activities. There is no age limit for osteotomy and patients should not be excluded from consideration based on chronologic age alone.[9,11] However, in these patients, the outcome can be poorer and the recovery longer.[12–14] Some conditions are correlated with a poorer prognosis, including (1) severe articular destruction (grade III Ahlbäck classification),[13,15] (2) patellofemoral arthrosis,[16] (4) joint instability, and (5) lateral tibial thrust.[14,16]

It should be noted that excessive malalignment may contraindicate HTO. For axis deviations exceeding 12° to 15°, a lateral closing wedge HTO would adversely tilt the tibial articular surface and would shorten the limb too much.[17] The medial collateral ligament must be checked that it is not injured (if it is, the surgeon should perform an opening wedge osteotomy instead).[18]

Therefore, the ideal candidate for an HTO is a young patient (<60 years of age), with isolated medial OA, with good range of motion, and without ligamentous instability.

PREOPERATIVE PLANNING

Preoperative planning is based on the preoperative imaging templating, which is performed using traditional templating methods and/or computer assistance to obtain the degree of angulation, the wedge size, and location of the osteotomy.

Essential radiographs include full-length standing alignment radiographs and standing anteroposterior and posteroanterior flexion view (Rosenberg view), as well as lateral and merchant views of the knee.[19,20]

In full-length standing radiographs, a line drawn from the center of the femoral head to the midpoint of the ankle joint represents the mechanical axis of the leg. A second line is drawn from the center of the femoral head to a point located at the junction of the medial two-thirds and the lateral one-third of the tibial plateau for varus gonarthrosis. A third line is drawn from the center of the ankle joint to the previous point. The angle formed by the intersection of the second and third lines determines the degree of correction required for realignment of the mechanical axis (**Fig. 1**). The goal is to calculate the angular correction necessary to produce 2° to 4° of mechanical or 8° to 10° of anatomic valgus.[6,8,21] When the angle of correction is obtained, different surgical techniques could be implemented to achieve it.

It is important to remember that in a normal healthy knee the weight force passes through the medial compartment.[22] It is considered normal to have a mechanical axis of 1° to 3° varus and an anatomic axis of 5° to 7° valgus. The weightbearing line should pass through the lateral 30% to 40% of the tibia plateau[22–25] (**Fig. 2**).

When treating unicompartmental medial gonarthrosis (in which the alignment is usually more than 10° off the normal range[26]) with valgus HTO, the goal is not to restore the physiologic alignment; it is, instead, to produce a slight valgus alignment to prevent recurring varus. Nearly 8° to 10° of valgus in the anatomic axis or 3° to 5° of valgus in the mechanical axis are considered optimal correction after surgery.[6,15,27–31] Slight varus correction can lead to recurrence of deformity, whereas overcorrection can cause lateral compartment osteoarthrosis.[15]

SURGICAL TECHNIQUE

LCWO is the conventional approach that was used by Coventry and colleagues[21] and Insall and colleagues[7] for varus gonarthrosis. Many minor modifications of the original Coventry technique of closing wedge osteotomy have occurred since the initial description. In many patients, arthroscopy can be performed before osteotomy to asses lateral compartment integrity and debride any degenerations.[32]

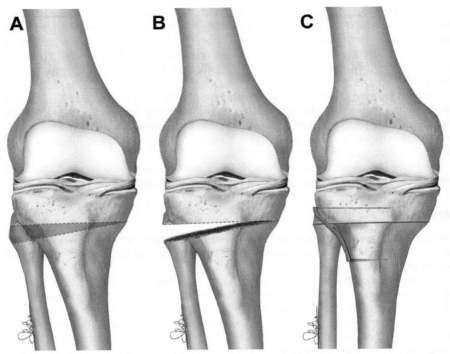

Fig. 1. LCWO. (*A*) Varus knee with bony cuts highlighted. (*B*) Removal of bony wedge from tibia and fibula. (*C*) Closing the gap and fixation using a Krakow staple.

The patient is positioned supine. A sandbag beneath the trochanteric region can help with placing the extremity in a neutral rotation. The knee is usually placed at 90° of flexion. Skin incision is then performed. The best results take place with a transverse incision running from fibular head toward tibial tubercle. This incision allows easy further TKA to be done.

In some patients, delicate isolation of the common peroneal nerve can be performed to prevent any possible nerve palsy caused by nerve entrapment in the osteotomy. Preoperative planning helps identify patients who will benefit from nerve isolation; for example, cases in which the nerve is near to the osteotomy line. The extensor muscles are carefully detached from the proximal tibia to expose the tibiofibular joint. The posterior tibia is subperiosteally exposed to allow insertion of a broad malleable retractor to protect neurovascular structures.

Under fluoroscopic control, a Kirschner wire is then inserted from lateral to medial parallel to the tibial joint line, at a distance of 2 to 2.5 cm from the joint line. A second wire is inserted obliquely, distally from the first wire at an angle that matches the correction planned, to restore the correct limb alignment.[18]

The angle of correction is quantitatively determined by the optimization of the lower limb mechanical axis. As suggested by Dugdale and colleagues,[8] the mechanical axis should be placed laterally at the 62% of tibial width. The wire is advanced obliquely to intersect with the first wire near medial tibial cortex.

With the wires used as guides, the osteotomy is then performed and the bone wedge extracted. The conformation of the bony wedge can be adjusted in the sagittal

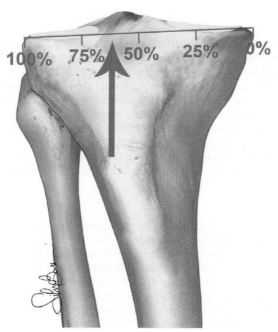

Fig. 2. Dugdale determined a point (*arrow*) located at 62% of the tibial plateau width when measured from the medial tibial plateau.

plane to correct flexion-extension deformity and tibial slope. This plane correction is a key point in the correction of a varus-valgus deformity combined with anteroposterior instability.[10,33] An intact medial periosteal wall is crucial to provide stability to the osteotomy because it acts as a fulcrum during the reduction maneuver.

Removal of a portion of the fibular head is then performed with a bony rongeur and the tibia is reduced. It is important to check the fibular head to ensure that it is in no way obstructing the complete osteotomy closure. Then mechanical realignment is verified using fluoroscopy.

Fixation can be accomplished in various ways, including cylinder cast only, external fixation, staple fixation, plate fixation, and fixed angle implants. More recently, however, calibrated cutting guides, rigid internal fixation devices, and early mobilization have been used in an effort to improve results and lower complication rates after LCWO.[34,35]

Importantly, if a fracture of the medial cortical occurs, a simple plate fixation is not enough to ensure the correct bone stability. In this case, it is mandatory to use locking compression plate fixation.

POSTOPERATIVE REGIMEN

Postoperative rehabilitation can be divided into 3 phases, each with different goals, with modifications based on the patient's general health, functional levels, and postoperative expectations.

The goal of the initial rehabilitation phase, during the 3 days of usual hospitalization, is to teach the patient how to independently move with appropriate walking aids and to learn exercises to be performed alone. For the first 6 weeks, partial weightbearing (15 kg) on crutches is allowed with maximum flexion restricted to 0° to 90°.[36] In the early phase, adequate analgesia is helpful to provide patient the ability of doing the exercises.

Before the intermediate phase, after 6 weeks, a control radiograph must be performed to check the bony union. If it is satisfactory, progressive weightbearing should be given. The brace can be weaned off to restore complete range of movement. Proprioceptive exercises are useful to improve muscle strength and patient awareness.

The late phase starts at 12 weeks after the osteotomy and full weightbearing should then be permitted. In case of an unsatisfactory union, physical therapies, such as electromagnetic pulsed fields and shockwaves, can be performed, paying attention to shortwave diathermy, which is contraindicated at the HTO site.

Within a year, the usual goal set in young patients is to be fit to return high-impact sports and be able to have an optimal proprioception and muscular strength.

RESULTS

The survival rate of HTO is influenced by correct patient selection, surgical technique, rigid fixation, and postoperative reabilitation.[37] The 10-year survival rates for closing wedge osteotomy reported in literature vary from 50% to 94.8% (**Table 1**).

Coventry and colleagues[21] also reported a 10-year delay in TKA in 75% of patients if an overcorrection to at least 8° of valgus was achieved.

The results of HTOs have been extensively studied and reported during the past 40 years. Insall,[38] Healy and Wilk[39] reviewed the experience of those first 3 decades (see **Table 1**).[17] Their main conclusions are following:

- After an HTO, pain recurs in most knees and most patients eventually will require a TKA.[41]
- Younger patients with moderate varus deformities achieve the best results. Obesity, undercorrection, and overcorrection are adverse factors.[41,46]
- The ideal correction is a femorotibial angle between 170° and 165°.
- The overall preoperative state of the knee is the most important determinant of an eventual good result.[47]
- Preoperative arthroscopic assessment of the knee is not useful.[48]
- Previous medial meniscectomy and anterior cruciate ligament (ACL) deficiency are not contraindications but previous lateral meniscectomy may be.[49]
- The addition of tibial tubercle elevation to the osteotomy in the case of associated patellofemoral arthritis is not necessary and it increases the complication rate.

Complications of Lateral Closing Wedge High Tibial Osteotomy

Complications of HTOs include recurrence of varus,[7,9] overcorrection and undercorrection,[7] altered patellofemoral kinematics (including patellar height changes),[50] patellofemoral malalignment,[51] increased quadriceps angle (Q-angle) and patellar subluxation, fractures, change in tibial inclination, increased joint line obliquity, delayed union and nonunion,[7] peroneal nerve and popliteal artery injury,[52] shortening of the leg, compartment syndrome, infection, and thromboembolism.

Duivenvoorden and colleagues[45] found the most common adverse event to be the need for hardware removal (48%), followed by the sensory palsy of the peroneal nerve (4%), and nonunion (2%). Multiple studies report a hardware removal rate of greater than 50%.[53–55] Severe adverse events were more common in patients with diabetes, active smoking, and displaced lateral hinge fractures, and in noncompliant patients.[56,57]

Table 1
The results of high tibial osteotomy

Study	Number of HTOs	Follow-up (y)	Results
Coventry et al,[21] 1993	87	3–14 (median 10)	87% survivorship at 5 y 66% survivorship at 10 y
Insall et al,[7] 1984	95	5–15 (mean 8.9)	85% good or excellent at 5 y 63% good or excellent at 9 y
Cass and Bryan,[40] 1988	86	≥5 (mean 9.1)	51% good 31 conversion to TKA
Matthews et al,[41] 1988	40	1–9	50% useful function at 5 y 28% useful function at 9 y 16 conversion to TKA
Sprenger and Doerzbacher,[42] 2003	76	Mean 10.8	86% survivorship at 5 y 74% survivorship at 10 y 56% survivorship at 15 y
Billings et al,[34] 2000	64	Average 8.5	85% survivorship at 5 y 53% survivorship at 10 y 21 conversion to TKA
Flecher et al,[13] 2006	301	12–28 (mean 18)	94.8% survivorship at 5 y 92.8% survivorship at 10 y 89.7% survivorship at 15 y 85.1% survivorship at 20 y 43 knees (14%) required revision
Yasuda et al,[43] 1992	56	6–15	88% satisfactory at 6 y 63% satisfactory at 10 y
Polat et al,[44] 2017	29	8–22	17% conversion to TKA 75% survivorship at 10 y
Duivenvoorden et al,[45] 2017	354	Mean 10	50% survivorship at 20 y

The advantages of closing wedge osteotomy compared with opening wedge osteotomy are a shorter consolidation times (7–8 weeks) and a natural tendency to decrease the tibial slope angle. The disadvantages are the risk of damaging the peroneal nerve and more variability in the obtained correction.

When the closing wedge HTO is compared with the unicompartmental knee arthroplasty, very-low-quality evidence shows no statistically significant differences between these 2 surgical treatments for medial compartmental knee OA.[58]

Performing TKA after HTO can be difficult because of valgus alignment, scarring of soft tissue with patella baja and bone stock, or anatomic changes in the proximal tibia.[58]

DISCUSSION

Realignment osteotomy of the knee continues to meet many of the original expectations. Although the current indications are relatively narrow, the surgeon should be confident in choosing corrective osteotomy when appropriate criteria are met. Long-term results linked with careful patient selection, accurate surgical technique, and appropriate postoperative alignment portray a favorable outlook for these procedures, particularly because the population at large is more active and is expected to have increasing longevity.[17]

The primary goals of a HTO are to reduce pain and to improve function. Furthermore, this procedure may slow down the OA process, consequently postponing knee arthroplasty, although results seem to deteriorate over time.[59]

Combined Anterior Cruciate Ligament Reconstruction and Closing Wedge High Tibial Osteotomy

It is possible to associate the osteotomy procedure with ligament reconstruction procedures. In complex patients presenting medial OA in varus knee with chronic ACL deficiency, it is possible to perform the HTO and the ACL reconstruction in a 1-stage procedure. Moreover the closing wedge osteotomy has the advantage of leaving the medial side of the proximal tibia untouched, making it easier to perform an ACL reconstruction using a hamstring tendons graft. Zaffagnini and colleagues[60] performed combined ACL reconstruction surgery and closing wedge HTO in varus knees with unicompartmental arthritis and chronic ACL deficiency. They obtained reduced pain and improved knee function, with an ACL revision rate of 6% and a progression in OA, in the medial compartment in 22% of subjects, with a mean of 6.5 years of follow-up.

A controversial topic concerning HTO is the role of posterior tibial slope and its effect on ACL-deficient knee. It is well known that HTO can alter the slope on purpose or inadvertently.[61] A multicentric study of the French Society of Orthopedic Surgery and Traumatology performed on 321 HTOs highlighted how opening wedge HTO increases the slope of a mean of 0.6°, whereas closing wedge HTO decreases slope of a mean of 0.7°.[62] The role of tibial slope is particularly interesting because it has been demonstrated that a steeper slope could be a risk factor for noncontact ACL lesions[63] caused by increased strain in the anteromedial bundle[64] due to the mechanism of anterior tibial translation when a compressive axial load is applied to knee joint.[65] The ability of a closing wedge HTO to reduce posterior tibial slope could possibly be beneficial in knees with ACL lesions.[60]

Combined Closing Wedge High Tibial Osteotomy and Meniscal Scaffold or Allograft Implant

The challenge of managing compromised joints such as unicompartmental OA is mainly based on the unfavorable articular environment. In fact, the cartilage layer is not the only tissue damaged at this stage of articular degeneration. The meniscus is often damaged as well, and knee alignment can also be altered. Correcting all joint abnormalities, such as instability, meniscus deficiency, and malalignment, is mandatory before addressing the damaged surface. Every attempt to regenerate meniscal or chondral tissues is doomed to failure if a correct alignment is not restored.[66,67] Marcacci and colleagues[68] obtained satisfactory results from combined realignment surgery and meniscal biological reconstruction with an improvement in subjective scores at 3-year follow-up. Younger patients reported a higher clinical and subjective improvement, showing again how conservative treatments could be a valid alternative to knee arthroplasty, especially in younger subjects.

SUMMARY

Valgus HTO is a technically challenging procedure but provides younger OA patients with a viable alternative to metal resurfacing while providing good to excellent results for return to physical activity. The lateral closing wedge approach has been demonstrated to be effective and to provide good to excellent results. It also can be associated with reconstructive surgeries for ligament and meniscal defect, which often are concomitant pathologic conditions with OA.

REFERENCES

1. Smith JO, Wilson AJ, Thomas NP. Osteotomy around the knee: evolution, principles and results. Knee Surg Sports Traumatol Arthrosc 2013;21(1):3–22.
2. Macewen W. 8th edition. Osteotomy, with an inquiry into the aetiology and pathology of knockknee, bow-leg and other osseous deformities of lower limbs, vol. 16. London (United Kingdom): I. and A. Churchill; 1880.
3. Putti V. Osteotomia ed Osteoclasia. La Chirurgia degli organi di movimento 1932; 17(1):7–35.
4. Putti V. Osteotomia ed Osteoclasia. In: Scientifiche Istituto Rizzoli, editor. Scritti Medici, vol. 2. Bologna (Italy): Scientifiche Istituto Rizzoli; 1952. p. 498–524.
5. Jackson J. Osteotomy for osteoarthritis of the knee. J Bone Joint Surg Br 1958;40: 826.
6. Coventry MB. Upper tibial osteotomy for osteoarthritis. J Bone Joint Surg Am 1985;67(7):1136–40.
7. Insall JN, Joseph DM, Msika C. High tibial osteotomy for varus gonarthrosis. A long-term follow-up study. J Bone Joint Surg Am 1984;66(7):1040–8.
8. Dugdale TW, Noyes FR, Styer D. Preoperative planning for high tibial osteotomy. The effect of lateral tibiofemoral separation and tibiofemoral length. Clin Orthop Relat Res 1992;(274):248–64.
9. Dowd GSE, Somayaji HS, Uthukuri M. High tibial osteotomy for medial compartment osteoarthritis. Knee 2006;13(2):87–92.
10. Noyes FR, Barber SD, Simon R. High tibial osteotomy and ligament reconstruction in varus angulated, anterior cruciate ligament-deficient knees. A two- to seven-year follow-up study. Am J Sports Med 1993;21(1):2–12.
11. Marti RK, Verhagen RA, Kerkhoffs GM, et al. Proximal tibial varus osteotomy. Indications, technique, and five to twenty-one-year results. J Bone Joint Surg Am 2001;83-A(2):164–70.
12. Gstöttner M, Michaela G, Pedross F, et al. Long-term outcome after high tibial osteotomy. Arch Orthop Trauma Surg 2008;128(1):111–5.
13. Flecher X, Parratte S, Aubaniac J-M, et al. A 12-28-year followup study of closing wedge high tibial osteotomy. Clin Orthop Relat Res 2006;452:91–6.
14. Naudie D, Bourne RB, Rorabeck CH, et al. The Insall Award. Survivorship of the high tibial valgus osteotomy. A 10- to -22-year followup study. Clin Orthop Relat Res 1999;(367):18–27.
15. Ivarsson I, Myrnerts R, Gillquist J. High tibial osteotomy for medial osteoarthritis of the knee. A 5 to 7 and 11 year follow-up. J Bone Joint Surg Br 1990;72(2): 238–44.
16. Rudan JF, Simurda MA. High tibial osteotomy. A prospective clinical and roentgenographic review. Clin Orthop Relat Res 1990;(255):251–6.
17. Insall JN, Scott WN. Insall & Scott surgery of the knee. New York: Elsevier Health Sciences; 2012.
18. Lobenhoffer P, van Heerwaarden RJ, Staubli AE, et al. High-tibial closed-wedge osteotomy. In: Osteotomies around the knee. Leipzig (Germany): AO Foundation Publishing. Thieme; 2008. p. 55–8.
19. Amendola A, Panarella L. High tibial osteotomy for the treatment of unicompartmental arthritis of the knee. Orthop Clin North Am 2005;36(4):497–504.

20. Christodoulou NA, Tsaknis RN, Sdrenias CV, et al. Improvement of proximal tibial osteotomy results by lateral retinacular release. Clin Orthop Relat Res 2005;441: 340–5.

21. Coventry MB, Ilstrup DM, Wallrichs SL. Proximal tibial osteotomy. A critical long-term study of eighty-seven cases. J Bone Joint Surg Am 1993;75(2):196–201.

22. Hsu RW, Himeno S, Coventry MB, et al. Normal axial alignment of the lower extremity and load-bearing distribution at the knee. Clin Orthop Relat Res 1990;(255):215–27.

23. Fujisawa Y, Masuhara K, Shiomi S. The effect of high tibial osteotomy on osteoarthritis of the knee. An arthroscopic study of 54 knee joints. Orthop Clin North Am 1979;10(3):585–608.

24. Moreland JR, Bassett LW, Hanker GJ. Radiographic analysis of the axial alignment of the lower extremity. J Bone Joint Surg Am 1987;69(5):745–9.

25. Tetsworth K, Paley D. Malalignment and degenerative arthropathy. Orthop Clin North Am 1994;25(3):367–77.

26. Iorio R, Healy WL. Unicompartmental arthritis of the knee. J Bone Joint Surg Am 2003;85-A(7):1351–64.

27. Hernigou P, Medevielle D, Debeyre J, et al. Proximal tibial osteotomy for osteoarthritis with varus deformity. A ten to thirteen-year follow-up study. J Bone Joint Surg Am 1987;69(3):332–54.

28. Engel GM, Lippert FG. Valgus tibial osteotomy: avoiding the pitfalls. Clin Orthop Relat Res 1981;(160):137–43.

29. Kettelkamp DB, Chao EY. A method for quantitative analysis of medial and lateral compression forces at the knee during standing. Clin Orthop Relat Res 1972;83: 202–13.

30. Koshino T, Morii T, Wada J, et al. High tibial osteotomy with fixation by a blade plate for medial compartment osteoarthritis of the knee. Orthop Clin North Am 1989;20(2):227–43.

31. Myrnerts R. Optimal correction in high tibial osteotomy for varus deformity. Acta Orthop Scand 1980;51(4):689–94.

32. Müller M, Strecker W. Arthroscopy prior to osteotomy around the knee? Arch Orthop Trauma Surg 2008;128(11):1217–21.

33. Preston C, Fulkerson E, Meislin R, et al. Osteotomy about the knee: applications, techniques, and results. J Knee Surg 2010;18(04):258–72.

34. Billings A, Scott DF, Camargo MP, et al. High tibial osteotomy with a calibrated osteotomy guide, rigid internal fixation, and early motion. Long-term follow-up. J Bone Joint Surg Am 2000;82(1):70–9.

35. Hofmann AA, Wyatt RW, Beck SW. High tibial osteotomy. Use of an osteotomy jig, rigid fixation, and early motion versus conventional surgical technique and cast immobilization. Clin Orthop Relat Res 1991;(271):212–7.

36. Aalderink KJ, Shaffer M, Amendola A. Rehabilitation following high tibial osteotomy. Clin Sports Med 2010;29(2):291–301.

37. Sherman C, Cabanela ME. Closing wedge osteotomy of the tibia and the femur in the treatment of gonarthrosis. Int Orthop 2010;34(2):173–84.

38. Insall JN. Osteotomy. In: Windsor RE, Insall JN, Scott WN, editors. Surgery of the knee. New York: Churchill Livingstone; 1993. p. 635–75.

39. Healy WL, Wilk RM. Osteotomy in treatment of the arthritic knee. In: Scott WN, editor. The knee.St. Louis (MO): Mosby; 1994. p. 1019–43.

40. Cass JR, Bryan RS. High tibial osteotomy. Clin Orthop Relat Res 1988;230:196–9.

41. Matthews LS, Goldstein SA, Malvitz TA, et al. Proximal tibial osteotomy. Factors that influence the duration of satisfactory function. Clin Orthop Relat Res 1988;(229):193–200.
42. Sprenger TR, Doerzbacher JF. Tibial osteotomy for the treatment of varus gonarthrosis. Survival and failure analysis to twenty-two years. J Bone Joint Surg Am 2003;85-A(3):469–74.
43. Yasuda K, Majima T, Tsuchida T, et al. A ten- to 15-year follow-up observation of high tibial osteotomy in medial compartment osteoarthrosis. Clin Orthop Relat Res 1992;(282):186–95.
44. Polat G, Balcı Hİ, Çakmak MF, et al. Long-term results and comparison of the three different high tibial osteotomy and fixation techniques in medial compartment arthrosis. J Orthop Surg Res 2017;12. https://doi.org/10.1186/s13018-017-0547-6.
45. Duivenvoorden T, van Diggele P, Reijman M, et al. Adverse events and survival after closing- and opening-wedge high tibial osteotomy: a comparative study of 412 patients. Knee Surg Sports Traumatol Arthrosc 2017;25(3):895–901.
46. Coventry MB. Osteotomy of the upper portion of the tibia for degenerative arthritis of the knee. A preliminary report. J Bone Joint Surg Am 1965;47:984–90.
47. Holden DL, James SL, Larson RL, et al. Proximal tibial osteotomy in patients who are fifty years old or less. A long-term follow-up study. J Bone Joint Surg Am 1988;70(7):977–82.
48. Keene JS, Monson DK, Roberts JM, et al. Evaluation of patients for high tibial osteotomy. Clin Orthop Relat Res 1989;(243):157–65.
49. Odenbring S, Tjörnstrand B, Egund N, et al. Function after tibial osteotomy for medial gonarthrosis below aged 50 years. Acta Orthop Scand 1989;60(5):527–31.
50. Scuderi GR, Windsor RE, Insall JN. Observations on patellar height after proximal tibial osteotomy. J Bone Joint Surg Am 1989;71(2):245–8.
51. Closkey RF, Windsor RE. Alterations in the patella after a high tibial or distal femoral osteotomy. Clin Orthop Relat Res 2001;(389):51–6.
52. Zaidi SH, Cobb AG, Bentley G. Danger to the popliteal artery in high tibial osteotomy. J Bone Joint Surg Br 1995;77(3):384–6.
53. Duivenvoorden T, Brouwer RW, Baan A, et al. Comparison of closing-wedge and opening-wedge high tibial osteotomy for medial compartment osteoarthritis of the knee: a randomized controlled trial with a six-year follow-up. J Bone Joint Surg Am 2014;96(17):1425–32.
54. Hoell S, Suttmoeller J, Stoll V, et al. The high tibial osteotomy, open versus closed wedge, a comparison of methods in 108 patients. Arch Orthop Trauma Surg 2005;125(9):638–43.
55. van Egmond N, van Grinsven S, van Loon CJM, et al. Better clinical results after closed- compared to open-wedge high tibial osteotomy in patients with medial knee osteoarthritis and varus leg alignment. Knee Surg Sports Traumatol Arthrosc 2016;24(1):34–41.
56. Martin R, Birmingham TB, Willits K, et al. Adverse event rates and classifications in medial opening wedge high tibial osteotomy. Am J Sports Med 2014;42(5):1118–26.
57. Sabzevari S, Ebrahimpour A, Roudi MK, et al. High tibial osteotomy: a systematic review and current concept. Arch Bone Jt Surg 2016;4(3):9.
58. Brouwer RW, Huizinga MR, Duivenvoorden T, et al. Osteotomy for treating knee osteoarthritis. Cochrane Database Syst Rev 2014;(12):CD004019.

59. Virolainen P, Aro HT. High tibial osteotomy for the treatment of osteoarthritis of the knee: a review of the literature and a meta-analysis of follow-up studies. Arch Orthop Trauma Surg 2004;124(4):258–61.

60. Zaffagnini S, Bonanzinga T, Grassi A, et al. Combined ACL reconstruction and closing-wedge HTO for varus angulated ACL-deficient knees. Knee Surg Sports Traumatol Arthrosc 2013;21(4):934–41.

61. Feucht MJ, Mauro CS, Brucker PU, et al. The role of the tibial slope in sustaining and treating anterior cruciate ligament injuries. Knee Surg Sports Traumatol Arthrosc 2013;21(1):134–45.

62. Ducat A, Sariali E, Lebel B, et al. Posterior tibial slope changes after opening- and closing-wedge high tibial osteotomy: a comparative prospective multicenter study. Orthop Traumatol Surg Res 2012;98(1):68–74.

63. Brandon ML, Haynes PT, Bonamo JR, et al. The association between posterior-inferior tibial slope and anterior cruciate ligament insufficiency. Arthroscopy 2006;22(8):894–9.

64. McLean SG, Oh YK, Palmer ML, et al. The relationship between anterior tibial acceleration, tibial slope, and ACL strain during a simulated jump landing task. J Bone Joint Surg Am 2011;93(14):1310–7.

65. Torzilli PA, Deng X, Warren RF. The effect of joint-compressive load and quadriceps muscle force on knee motion in the intact and anterior cruciate ligament-sectioned knee. Am J Sports Med 1994;22(1):105–12.

66. Gomoll AH, Filardo G, Almqvist FK, et al. Surgical treatment for early osteoarthritis. Part II: allografts and concurrent procedures. Knee Surg Sports Traumatol Arthrosc 2012;20(3):468–86.

67. Heijink A, Gomoll AH, Madry H, et al. Biomechanical considerations in the pathogenesis of osteoarthritis of the knee. Knee Surg Sports Traumatol Arthrosc 2012; 20(3):423–35.

68. Marcacci M, Zaffagnini S, Kon E, et al. Unicompartmental osteoarthritis: an integrated biomechanical and biological approach as alternative to metal resurfacing. Knee Surg Sports Traumatol Arthrosc 2013;21(11):2509–17.

Distal Femoral Osteotomy and Lateral Meniscus Allograft Transplant

Natalie L. Leong, MD[a,b,]*, Taylor M. Southworth, BS[c],
Brian J. Cole, MD, MBA[d,e]

KEYWORDS

- Distal femoral osteotomy • Lateral meniscus allograft transplant • Valgus knee

KEY POINTS

- Patient selection is critical for performing combined lateral meniscus allograft transplant (LMAT) and distal femoral osteotomy (DFO).
- Preoperative expectation setting and counseling regarding postrehabilitation are extremely important to preparing patients for surgery and recovery.
- When performing a combined DFO/LMAT, the senior author (BJC) typically first performs the meniscal transplant and then the osteotomy.
- Although the literature suggests that patients improve significantly after this procedure in terms of functional outcomes, the number of patients studied has been limited to date.

INTRODUCTION

Distal femoral varus-producing osteotomy can be performed in the setting of lateral meniscal transplant (LMAT) to correct valgus malalignment of the knee and thus offload the lateral compartment.[1] Compared with the combination of high tibial osteotomy and medial meniscus transplant, DFO and LMAT are far less commonly performed, due to the lower incidence of valgus-malaligned knees. Over time, the incidence of osteotomies in North America had declined in light of more reliable and predictable arthroplasty solutions for younger and middle-aged patients with knee arthrosis.[2] With advances in biologic restoration and the use of cartilage restoration techniques, however, osteotomies are becoming increasingly popular, especially in

Disclosure Statement: The authors have nothing to disclose.
[a] Department of Orthopaedic Surgery, University of Maryland, Baltimore, 2200 Kernan Drive, Baltimore, MD 21207, USA; [b] Veterans Affairs Maryland Healthcare System, Baltimore, MD, USA; [c] Department of Orthopaedic Surgery, Rush University Medical Center, 1611 West Harrison, Suite 300, Chicago, IL 60612, USA; [d] Department of Orthopedics, Rush University Medical Center, 1611 West Harrison, Suite 300, Chicago, IL 60612, USA; [e] Department of Surgery, Rush Oak Park Hospital, 1611 West Harrison, Suite 300, Chicago, IL 60612, USA
* Corresponding author. 110 S. Paca Street, 6th Floor, Baltimore, MD 21201.
E-mail address: nleong@som.umaryland.edu

Clin Sports Med 38 (2019) 387–399
https://doi.org/10.1016/j.csm.2019.02.007
0278-5919/19/Published by Elsevier Inc.
sportsmed.theclinics.com

younger patients.[2] In these surgeries, it is important to address all knee joint comorbidities, including meniscal deficiency, chondral and osteochondral defects, and ligamentous insufficiency. A failure to correct these comorbidities can result in incomplete relief of symptoms and suboptimal outcomes.

Two techniques have been used to correct valgus: medial closing wedge osteotomy and lateral opening wedge osteotomy. The advantages of the opening wedge technique over the medial closing wedge technique include a single bone cut, avoidance of vascular structures, and theoretically better control of the amount of correction.[2,3] Disadvantages include the risk for delayed union or nonunion given that 2 bone-graft interfaces must heal and irritation of sensitive lateral knee structures by hardware or surgical trauma.[2] With these considerations in mind, the senior author's (BJC) preference is lateral opening DFO.[4]

LMAT is often indicated in a younger patient with meniscal deficiency after meniscectomy. Load that is transmitted through the medial and lateral compartments of the knee is shared between the menisci and the articular cartilage; on the medial side the load is shared evenly between these 2 components. The lateral meniscus, however, covers approximately 50% of the lateral tibial plateau and carries 70% of the load transmitted across the lateral compartment of the knee. Thus, the lateral compartment is more meniscal dependent than the medial compartment.[5]

This article reviews the indications, preoperative considerations, technique, postoperative rehabilitative protocol, and results in the literature associated with concurrent varus-producing DFO and LMAT.

INDICATIONS

Careful patient selection is critical to the success of distal femoral osteotomy and lateral meniscus allograft transplant. Although the decision to proceed to surgery can vary according to a variety of patient factors, **Table 1** presents the general indications and contraindications to performing distal femoral with LMAT.

PREOPERATIVE PLANNING

- Physical examination
  - Inspection
  - Alignment (Q angle)
  - Muscle bulk
  - Prior surgical incisions
  - Palpation
  - Tenderness

Table 1
The general indications and contraindications to performing distal femoral with lateral meniscal transplant

Indications	Contraindications
• Age <60 y old	• Tricompartmental arthritis
• Symptomatic unicompartmental arthritis	• Inflammatory arthritis
• Malalignment with or without cartilage deficiency	• Medial compartment articular surface pathology
• Malalignment with lateral meniscal deficiency	• Baseline knee flexion <90°
• Normal, or correctable, ligamentous status	• Flexion contracture >10°
• Willingness to comply with rehabilitation	• Medial/lateral tibial subluxation >1 cm
	• Body mass index >35 kg/m²

- ○ Crepitus (medial, lateral, patellofemoral)
- ○ Active and passive range of motion
  - ▪ Hip
  - ▪ Knee
- ○ Strength
  - ▪ Core
  - ▪ Lower extremity
- ○ Flexibility
- ○ Ober test
- ○ Hamstring
- ○ Neurovascular examination
  - ▪ Bilateral lower extremity
- ○ Patellar examination
  - ▪ Tilt
  - ▪ Apprehension
  - ▪ J sign
  - ▪ Static and dynamic Q-angle assessment
  - ▪ Crepitus
- ○ Knee tests of stability and special tests
  - ▪ Pivot shift, Lachman, anterior drawer
  - ▪ Posterior drawer
  - ▪ Varus and valgus stress (at full extension and at 30° of flexion)
- • Imaging (**Fig. 1**)
  - ○ Standard weight-bearing radiographic series

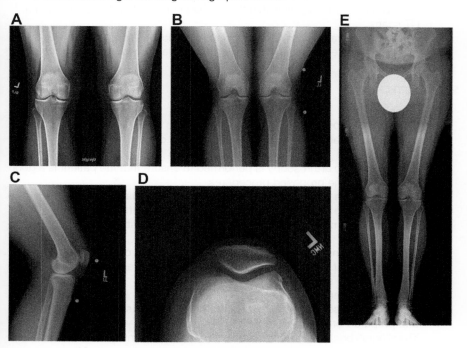

Fig. 1. Standard knee radiograph series demonstrating left knee valgus alignment, mild lateral compartment narrowing, and flattening of the condyle in a 25-year-old female patient: (A) AP, (B) Rosenberg, (C) lateral, (D) Merchant, and (E) standing long-leg alignment.

- Anteroposterior (AP), Rosenberg, lateral, and Merchant views
- Used to evaluate joint degeneration and overall alignment
- Standardized sizing AP radiographs are performed weight bearing with the knees flexed 45° and the beam angled 10° in the caudal direction.
- A calibration marker is placed at the level of the joint on the affected side.
  o Long-leg alignment views
    - Measurements of the mechanical axis are documented on the long-leg radiographs.
    - Lateral non–weight bearing
    - Sizing radiograph performed with the markers placed at the level of the patella and the joint line.
  o MRI
    - Used to evaluate the soft tissues of the knee and the presence or absence of soft tissue fluid or joint effusion.
    - The articular cartilage, menisci, and ligaments should be closely evaluated.
    - Unicompartmental bone edema can be an indicator of chronic compartment overload.
    - Meniscal volume can be assessed using the coronal and sagittal sequences; however, caution should be used in evaluating meniscal injury after a prior meniscal surgery.
    - Gradient-echo sequences are used to decipher articular cartilage from the surrounding joint fluid and subchondral bone; however, gradient-echo sequences are not able to identify intrasubstance cartilage defects.
    - T2-weighted or short tau inversion recovery fluid sequences are used to evaluate internal signal within the cartilage or subchondral bone edema.
  o CT scans
    - Helpful adjuvant in cases of prior anterior cruciate ligament reconstructions in which there is concern for bone tunnel enlargement

SURGICAL TECHNIQUE

- Positioning
  o The patient is positioned supine on the operative table with a lateral post, and a tourniquet is placed over the thigh and inflated during the case.
- Arthroscopy
  o First, diagnostic arthroscopy is performed to ensure that the patient is a good candidate for the proposed procedures.
  o Specifically, the anterolateral and anteromedial standard portals are used to confirm that the lateral meniscus is deficient or absent.
  o Any remaining native lateral meniscus is removed with a No. 11 blade and shaver (**Fig. 2**).
  o It is then confirmed that there is no significant cartilage deficiency in the medial compartment. If there is a lateral femoral condyle defect (**Fig. 3**), that can be addressed with a concurrent osteochondral allograft.
- Meniscus transplant
  o Once the meniscus deficiency is confirmed, the meniscal allograft is thawed and prepared on the back table (**Fig. 4**).
  o The allograft bone bridge is prepared with a slot that is 8 mm wide and 8 mm deep.
  o A polypropylene suture is placed in the posterolateral corner of the meniscus.
  o A slot is made for the LMAT that is 1 cm deep and 8 mm wide, in line with the patellar tendon and anterior and posterior horns (**Fig. 5**). First, a trough is

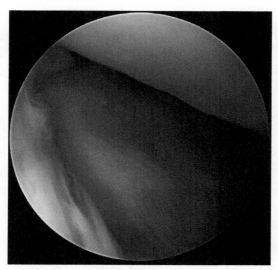

Fig. 2. Deficient meniscus in a 25-year-old woman

established using a bone-cutting shaver with valgus stress on the knee. Then, the hook and drill guide are used to place a guide pin, over which an 8-mm reamer is used to ream the slot. The remaining bone is removed using a pituitary rongeur, and an 8-mm box cutter rasp is used to finish the slot.

○ The lateral knee is marked in preparation for the meniscal transplant and the DFO (**Fig. 6**).

○ A curvilinear incision one-third above the joint line and two-thirds below the joint line is then made on the lateral side of the knee, between the iliotibial band and the biceps femoris, elevating the lateral head of the gastrocnemius (**Fig. 7**A).

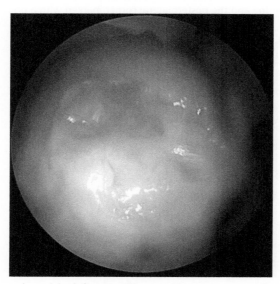

Fig. 3. Lateral femoral condyle defect in a 25-year-old woman, measuring 18 mm × 18 mm.

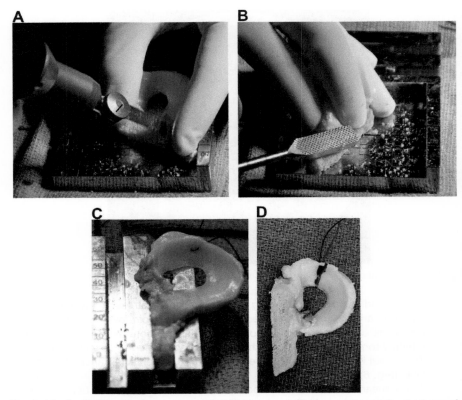

Fig. 4. Meniscal allograft preparation. (*A*) Utilizing an oscillating saw to create an appropriately sized bone bridge. (*B*) Trimming the sides of the bone bridge of the graft. (*C*) Graft within sizing device. (*D*) Final meniscal allograft after preparation with an 8-mm wide and 8-mm deep bone bridge and the posterolateral corner marked with a polypropylene suture.

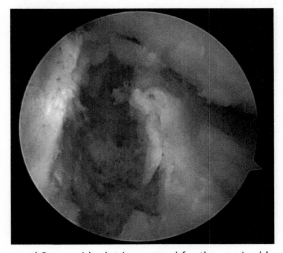

Fig. 5. A 1-cm deep and 8-mm wide slot is prepared for the meniscal bone bridge.

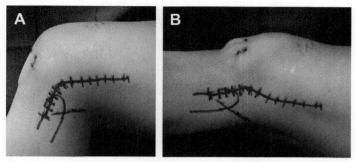

Fig. 6. The lateral knee is marked in preparation for the meniscal transplant and the DFO.

- ○ The prepared lateral meniscus allograft is then introduced into the into the lateral compartment via the arthrotomy with the help of a long, flexible nitinol suture passing pin (see **Fig. 7**B).
- ○ The meniscus allograft is secured within the tibial slot using a bioabsorbable cortical interference screw and within the capsule with a series of inside-out sutures.
- ○ Direct suture of the anterior horn through the incision with 1 Vicryl is also performed.
- Osteochondral allograft
  - ○ After fixing the meniscus, an osteochondral allograft is performed to the lateral femoral condyle if necessary.
  - ○ For the osteochondral allograft, the arthrotomy is extended approximately 4 cm.
  - ○ The sizing tubes are used to determine the size of transplant, and the defect is cored to 8 mm in depth.
  - ○ The defect is then measured at the 12 o'clock, 3 o'clock, 6 o'clock, and 9 o'clock positions and irrigated thoroughly with pulse lavage.

An osteochondral allograft is then irrigated well with the pulse lavage to remove any marrow elements and gently impacted into place.

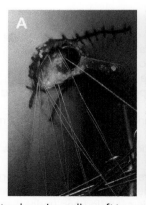
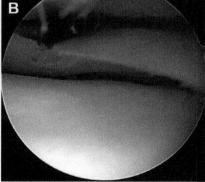

Fig. 7. Lateral meniscus allograft transplant. (*A*) A curvilinear incision is made one-third above and two-thirds below the joint line, posterior to the lateral collateral ligament. (*B*) The lateral meniscus allograft is introduced into the lateral compartment using the polypropylene suture.

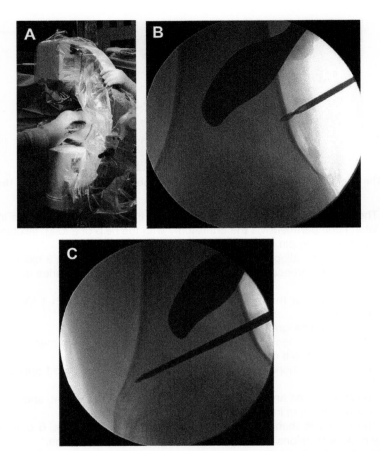

Fig. 8. (*A*) An AP view of the distal femur is obtained intraoperatively using a large C-arm. (*B*) A Kirschner wire is placed at the site of the planned osteotomy. (*C*) A second parallel Kirschner wires are inserted at the level of the planned osteotomy, and together, the 2 wires will serve as a template for the osteotomy.

- DFO
  - Next, the incision is extended proximally on the lateral side of the knee to approximately 10 cm proximal of the lateral femoral epicondyle.
  - The subcutaneous tissues are dissected to the iliotibial band.
  - The iliotibial band is incised in line with the skin incision.
  - Care is taken to incise only the tendinous portion of the iliotibial band and not the vastus musculature deep to it.
  - The vastus lateralis is bluntly elevated anteriorly off the posterior intermuscular septum.
  - Cautery is used to coagulate any large femoral perforating vessels as they are encountered.
  - Once the distal femur is exposed, retractors are carefully placed anteriorly and posteriorly to protect the soft tissue and neurovascular bundle, respectively.
  - Once the exposure is complete, the knee is extended and under fluoroscopic guidance a guidewire is inserted mirroring the trajectory of the osteotomy (**Fig. 8**).

○ The appropriate guide wire starting position is 2 cm proximal to the lateral epi-
condyle, aiming distally toward to proximal aspect of the medial epicondyle.
○ A second guide wire is placed parallel to the first (see **Fig. 8**C).
○ Placed a locking plate with three 6.5mm screws distally and four 4.5mm bicort-
ical screws proximally. They were viewed under direct fluoroscopy.
○ A small oscillating saw is used to initiate the osteotomy on the lateral cortex.
○ Cutting proximal to the parallel pins, further from the joint surface, decreases the
likelihood of stress-riser propagation into the trochlea or through the medial cortex.
○ The saw is followed by osteotomes in stacked fashion to a depth 1 cm from the
medial cortex.
○ Calibrated anterior and posterior wedges are placed to the planned preopera-
tive level of correction.
○ The wedge position is assessed.
○ The anterior wedge is removed and the plate is placed in the osteotomy site
and secured with sequential screws.
○ Under fluoroscopic guidance, care should be taken to ensure the plate wedge
is securely in the osteotomy site (**Fig. 9**).
○ Cortical and cancellous allograft can be used in the osteotomy site.
○ The tourniquet is released and hemostasis is achieved.
○ The wound is then irrigated and closed in a standard layered fashion

At the conclusion of the sterile dressing, patients have a cooling unit incorporated into
the dressing and a hinged knee brace locked in extension placed on the operative leg.

POSTOPERATIVE REGIMEN

The postoperative protocol shown in **Table 2** is used by the senior author (BJC) after
combined DFO and lateral meniscus allograft transplant.

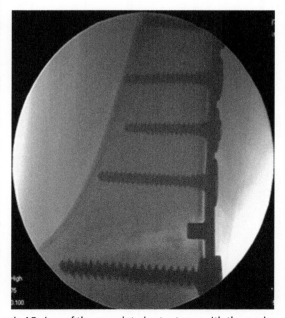

Fig. 9. A fluoroscopic AP view of the completed osteotomy with the wedge and plate in place.

Table 2
Postoperative protocol for concurrent lateral meniscal allograft transplant and distal femoral osteotomy

Phase	Weight-Bearing	Brace	Range of Motion	Exercises
I (0–2 wk)	Heel touch	Locked in full extension at all times[a] Off for hygiene and home exercise only	Gentle passive 0°–90° Continuous passive motion machine 0°–90°	Heel slides, quad sets, patellar mobs, straight leg raise, calf pumps at home
II (2–8 wk)	2–6 wk: heel touch 6–8 wk: advance 25% weekly until full	2–6 wk: locked 0°–90° Discontinue brace at 6 wk	Advance as tolerated with caution during flexion >90° to protect post horn of meniscus	2–6 wk: add side-lying hip and core, advance quad set, and stretching[b] 6–8 wk: addition of heel raises, total gym (closed chain), gait normalization, eccentric quads, eccentric hamstrings Advance core, glutes, and pelvic stability
III (8–12 wk)	Full	None	Full	Progress closed chain activities Advance hamstring work, lunges/leg press 0°–90° only proprioception/balance exercises Begin stationary bike
IV (12–24 wk)	Full	None	Full	Progress phase III exercises and functional activities: walking lunges, planks, bridges, exercise Ball, half exercise Ball Advance core/glutes and balance
V (6–9 mo)	Full	None	Full	Advance all activity, such as running, jumping, pivoting, and sports, until cleared by surgeon

[a] Brace may be removed for sleeping after first postoperative visit (days 7–14).
[b] Avoid any tibial rotation for 8 wk to protect meniscus.

At the authors' institution, this procedure is performed as an outpatient procedure. Because these procedures can be lengthy; however, an overnight stay is reasonable.

RESULTS

There is a paucity of studies that address the outcomes of combined LMAT and DFO. In 1997, Cameron and Saha[6] reported on 63 patients who underwent meniscal allograft transplant, of whom 6 had a DFO as well. In this cohort, 2 patients were noted to have an excellent outcome, 3 patients had a good outcome, and 1 patient had a poor outcome, and there was an improvement in knee score and activity scale.[6] More recently, Cameron and colleagues[2] reported a series of 31 patients who underwent lateral distal femoral opening wedge osteotomies, but only 2 of the patients underwent a combined procedure LMAT. Similarly, Verdonk and colleagues[7] reported on 61 patients who underwent LMAT, but only 2 of these patients underwent a DFO as well. Gomoll and colleagues[8] reported on 7 patients who underwent osteotomy, meniscal transplant, and osteochondral allograft, of whom 2 had lateral-sided procedures. In general, these studies that included patients who underwent DFO and LMAT in their cohorts reported improved functional outcome scores and return to physical activities, but the scarcity of patients makes it difficult to make quantitative statements regarding the outcomes of this procedure.

Although reports on the outcomes after combined LMAT and DFO are limited, there exists plenty of literature that assesses the midterm and long-term outcome of varus-producing DFO for valgus knees.[2,9–12] Varus-producing DFO for valgus knees has a reported success rate ranging from 64% to 82% at 10 years after surgery but only 45% by 15 years after surgery.[13] The long-term survival of an isolated DFO has been reported to be 91% at 8 years[9] and 64% to 87% at 10 years.[10,14,15] These studies should be interpreted, however, with the understanding that a majority of these studies examine varus-producing DFO in the setting of unicompartmental arthritis rather than in the context of knee preservation with meniscus transplant and the treatment of more focal defects in articular cartilage.

With regard to meniscal transplant, it has been shown that functional outcome scores improved after the procedure, and there was no difference whether a concurrent osteotomy was performed.[16–18] There has been some ambiguity in the literature regarding whether outcomes are different for LMAT and medial meniscal allograft transplant (MMAT). At short-term follow-up, it has been the authors' experience that there is no difference in the survival between LMAT and MMAT, with a reoperation rate of 32% and an allograft survival rate of more than 95% at a minimum of 2-year follow-up.[19] Parkinson and colleagues[20] reported a significantly higher 89% survival rate of LMAT at 5 years compared with 62% for MMAT. Conversely, Hommen and colleagues[21] reported a 50% failure rate for LMAT at 10 years compared with a 25% failure rate for MMAT. This wide variation in outcomes reported in the literature may be due to differences in surgical technique, patient population, and follow-up duration.

SUMMARY

Patients presenting with lateral meniscus insufficiency and valgus malalignment can be a formidable treatment challenge. Good results have been reported with several established treatment options, including injections, bracing, osteotomy, and arthroplasty.[8] A combined DFO and LMAT represents a good option for younger patients looking to avoid knee arthroplasty and the activity limitations associated with arthroplasty. To ensure an optimal outcome, patient selection and preoperative counseling and expectation setting are of the utmost importance. In this article, the senior author's (BJC) preferred technique for performing DFO and LMAT is presented as well as a recommended postoperative protocol and a summary of results found in the literature. There is a need to better define outcomes after concurrent DFO and LMAT, but achieving sufficient sample size represents a challenge, given the relative rarity of this procedure.

REFERENCES

1. Harris JD, Hussey K, Saltzman BM, et al. Cartilage repair with or without meniscal transplantation and osteotomy for lateral compartment chondral defects of the knee: case series with minimum 2-year follow-up. Orthop J Sports Med 2014; 2(10). 2325967114551528.
2. Cameron JI, McCauley JC, Kermanshahi AY, et al. Lateral opening-wedge distal femoral osteotomy: pain relief, functional improvement, and survivorship at 5 years. Clin Orthop Relat Res 2015;473(6):2009–15.
3. Görtz S, Bugbee W. Valgus malalignment: diagnosis, osteotomy techniques, clinical outcomes. Philadelphia: Elsevier Saunders; 2008. p. 896–904.
4. Gitelis ME, Weber AE, Yanke AB, et al. Distal femoral osteotomy. In: Miller MD, Cole BJ, editors. Operative techniques: knee surgery. Philadelphia: Elsevier; 2017. p. 144–51.
5. Amendola A. Knee osteotomy and meniscal transplantation: indications, technical considerations, and results. Sports Med Arthrosc Rev 2007;15(1):32–8.
6. Cameron JC, Saha S. Meniscal allograft transplantation for unicompartmental arthritis of the knee. Clin Orthop Relat Res 1997;337:164–71.
7. Verdonk PC, Demurie A, Almqvist KF, et al. Transplantation of viable meniscal allograft. Survivorship analysis and clinical outcome of one hundred cases. J Bone Joint Surg Am 2005;87(4):715–24.
8. Gomoll AH, Kang RW, Chen AL, et al. Triad of cartilage restoration for unicompartmental arthritis treatment in young patients: meniscus allograft transplantation, cartilage repair and osteotomy. J Knee Surg 2009;22(2):137–41.
9. Zarrouk A, Bouzidi R, Karray B, et al. Distal femoral varus osteotomy outcome: is associated femoropatellar osteoarthritis consequential? Orthop Traumatol Surg Res 2010;96(6):632–6.
10. Wang JW, Hsu CC. Distal femoral varus osteotomy for osteoarthritis of the knee. J Bone Joint Surg Am 2005;87(1):127–33.
11. Thein R, Bronak S, Haviv B. Distal femoral osteotomy for valgus arthritic knees. J Orthop Sci 2012;17(6):745–9.
12. O'Malley MP, Pareek A, Reardon PJ, et al. Distal femoral osteotomy: lateral opening wedge technique. Arthrosc Tech 2016;5(4):e725–30.
13. Backstein D, Morag G, Hanna S, et al. Long-term follow-up of distal femoral varus osteotomy of the knee. J Arthroplasty 2007;22(4 Suppl 1):2–6.
14. Finkelstein JA, Gross AE, Davis A. Varus osteotomy of the distal part of the femur. A survivorship analysis. J Bone Joint Surg Am 1996;78(9):1348–52.
15. Ekeland A, Nerhus TK, Dimmen S, et al. Good functional results of distal femoral opening-wedge osteotomy of knees with lateral osteoarthritis. Knee Surg Sports Traumatol Arthrosc 2016;24(5):1702–9.
16. Koh YG, Kim YS, Kwon OR, et al. Comparative matched-pair analysis of keyhole bone-plug technique versus arthroscopic-assisted pullout suture technique for lateral meniscal allograft transplantation. Arthroscopy 2018;34(6): 1940–7.

17. LaPrade RF, Wills NJ, Spiridonov SI, et al. A prospective outcomes study of meniscal allograft transplantation. Am J Sports Med 2010;38(9):1804–12.
18. Lee BS, Kim HJ, Lee CR, et al. Clinical outcomes of meniscal allograft transplantation with or without other procedures: a systematic review and meta-analysis. Am J Sports Med 2018;46(12):3047–56.
19. McCormick F, Harris JD, Abrams GD, et al. Survival and reoperation rates after meniscal allograft transplantation: analysis of failures for 172 consecutive transplants at a minimum 2-year follow-up. Am J Sports Med 2014;42(4):892–7.
20. Parkinson B, Smith N, Asplin L, et al. Factors Predicting Meniscal Allograft Transplantation Failure. Orthop J Sports Med 2016;4(8). 2325967116663185.
21. Hommen JP, Applegate GR, Del Pizzo W. Meniscus allograft transplantation: ten-year results of cryopreserved allografts. Arthroscopy 2007;23(4):388–93.

High Tibial Osteotomy and Medial Meniscus Transplant

Joseph N. Liu, MD[a], Avinesh Agarwalla, MD[b], Andreas H. Gomoll, MD[c],*

KEYWORDS

- High tibial osteotomy • Medial meniscal transplant • Meniscal deficiency
- Varus malalignment

KEY POINTS

- High tibial osteotomy is preferred in younger, more active patients and has been shown to be the most cost-effective treatment modality in this population.
- Meniscal allograft transplant with or without concomitant cartilage procedures is also performed in young, active patients with meniscal deficiency.
- Opening-wedge high tibial osteotomy is preferred over the closing-wedge technique due to reduced technical difficulty, better survival, and theoretic advantages in conversion to arthroplasty.
- Outcomes following high tibial osteotomy with concomitant medial meniscal transplant are lacking due to the rarity of the procedure.

INTRODUCTION

In older patients with isolated medial compartment arthritis and varus deformity, total knee arthroplasty and unicompartmental knee arthroplasty provide adequate pain relief and excellent outcomes. The proportion of patients younger than 55 years receiving a total knee arthroplasty increased by 40% from 2002 to 2007.[1] This patient population expects to perform better in activities of daily living, work, and leisure, often at higher levels of demand.[2] However, in younger, more active patients, there are concerns of a higher risk of prosthesis wear, which may result in a higher risk of failure and subsequent revision. High tibial osteotomy (HTO) is an alternative treatment modality in young, active patients with isolated medial compartment osteoarthritis.[3–5] Following an HTO, patients demonstrate reduced pain, improved function, and a slowing of knee deterioration, thereby reducing the necessity of knee arthroplasty.[6] Furthermore, HTO is a cost-effective treatment alternative than knee arthroplasty in younger patients.[7]

Disclosure Statement: The authors do not have any financial disclosures that directly impact the content of this article.
[a] Department of Orthopedic Surgery, Loma Linda Medical Center, 11234 Anderson Street, Loma Linda, CA, USA; [b] Department of Orthopaedic Surgery, Westchester Medical Center, 100 Woods Road, Valhalla, NY 10595, USA; [c] Division of Sports Medicine, Department of Orthopedic Surgery, Hospital for Special Surgery, 535 East 70th Street, New York, NY 10021, USA
* Corresponding author.
E-mail address: gomolloffice@hss.edu

Despite an improvement in functional outcome scores, patient satisfaction, as well as procedural survivorship,[8–11] the incidence of osteotomies has declined in North America in lieu of arthroplasty solutions in younger patients with knee arthrosis.[12–14] However, due to improvements in meniscal and cartilage restoration techniques, there is renewed interest in knee osteotomies in young patients with knee pain and joint surface defects.[15] Meniscal allograft transplant (MAT) is often indicated in young, active patients with total or subtotal meniscal damage.[16] Lateral MAT is more commonly performed than medial MAT due to a higher incidence of osteoarthritis in the lateral compartment.[17] The lateral meniscus functions in stress protection and load sharing of the lateral compartment, whereas the medial meniscus is also a secondary stabilizer of the knee.[18–20] Medial meniscal allograft transplantation results in good pain relief, functional improvement, and prolonged clinical and radiographic survival.[21,22] However, at long-term follow-up (>10 years), 52.6% and 56.6% of medial and lateral MATs survive, with lateral MATs demonstrating greater pain relief and functional improvement.[23] It is important to note that a synergistic relationship likely exists between knee realignment and cartilage restoration. Improvement in the mechanical axis provides improved cartilage healing, whereas an improvement in the cartilage status provides increased pain relief following HTO.[5,24,25]

This article reviews the indications, preoperative considerations, technique, and postoperative rehabilitative protocol, as well as outcomes associated with HTO with concomitant medial MAT.

INDICATIONS

The decision to proceed with operative management is dependent on individual patient needs and benefits to optimize patient outcomes following HTO with concomitant medial MAT. The general indications and contraindications to performing HTO with concomitant medial MAT is provided in **Table 1**.[26–30]

OPENING-WEDGE VERSUS CLOSING-WEDGE OSTEOTOMY

The lateral closing-wedge HTO was traditionally more common; however, the medial opening-wedge HTO has become increasingly more popular as an alternative treatment modality.[31] The opening-wedge HTO provides several theoretic advantages over the closing-wedge technique. These advantages include an easier and potentially more precise correction of the deformity, preservation of the proximal tibial bone stock,

Table 1	
General indications and contraindications to performing high tibial osteotomy with concomitant medial meniscal allograft transplant	
Indications	**Contraindications**
• Age < 60 years	• Established osteoarthritis (>50% joint space loss)
• Symptomatic medial compartment overload	• Significant chondrosis in lateral compartment
• Medial joint line pain	• Deformity >15°
• Varus malalignment	• Inflammatory arthritis
• Medial meniscal deficiency	• Lateral meniscal deficiency
• Normal, or correctable, ligamentous integrity	• Baseline knee flexion <90°
• Willing to comply with rehabilitation protocol	• Flexion contracture >10°
• Focal cartilage defects can be present	• Medial/lateral tibial subluxation >1 cm
	• Body mass index >35 kg/m^2
	• Open growth plates

protection of the proximal tibiofemoral joint, protection of the peroneal nerve, as well as a reduced incidence of compartment syndrome.[31] Furthermore, due to preservation of proximal bone stock, the opening-wedge HTO provides fewer technical issues during conversion to total knee arthroplasty than the closing-wedge technique.[32] Despite these theoretic advantages, there is no difference in functional outcome or the duration of maximal improvement between either technique.[33] Although the opening-wedge HTO results in a higher rate of adverse events, it results in a better survival rate than the closing-wedge technique.[34] Because of reduced technical difficulty, better survival, as well as theoretic advantages in conversion to total knee arthroplasty, the senior author (AHG) prefers the opening-wedge technique.

PREOPERATIVE PLANNING

- Physical examination
  - Inspection
    - Prior surgical incisions
  - Palpation
    - Medial and lateral compartment
    - Tenderness
    - Crepitus
    - Muscle bulk
  - Mechanical axis alignment
  - Active and passive range of motion
    - Hip
    - Knee
  - Strength
    - Core
    - Bilateral lower extremity
  - Flexibility
  - Patellar examination
    - Tilt
    - Apprehension
    - Crepitus
    - J-sign
    - Static and dynamic Q-angle assessment
  - Ligamentous stability assessment
    - Cruciate ligaments
      - Pivot shift, Lachman, anterior drawer, posterior drawer
    - Collateral ligaments
      - Varus and valgus stress
        - Performed at full extension and 30° flexion
  - Neurovascular examination
- Diagnostic imaging
  - Radiographs
    - Standard weight-bearing radiographic series
      - Evaluate joint degeneration and alignment
      - Anteroposterior (AP), Rosenberg, lateral, and Merchant views
        - AP Rosenberg radiograph performed in standard weight-bearing fashion with knee flexed to 45° and beam angled 10° in the caudal direction. Rosenberg view evaluates amount of posterior femoral wear in flexion.

- o Lateral radiograph to evaluate posterior tibial slope. HTO has been shown to impact the degree of tibial slope.[26]
- o Additional radiographs may be obtained depending on suspicion of concomitant ligamentous injuries:
  - Anterior cruciate ligament (ACL): no additional views.
  - Posterior cruciate ligament: bilateral kneeling posterior stress radiograph.[27]
  - Posterolateral corner: varus stress radiograph performed at 20° and 30° of flexion.[35]
- Long-leg alignment view
  - Bilateral weight-bearing hip-knee-ankle radiographs are obtained to evaluate mechanical axis.
    - o Calculated as a percentage of width across the tibial plateau.
    - o Medial border is considered 0% and lateral border is considered 100%.
    - o Varus malalignment occurs when the mechanical axis is medial to the apex of the medial tibial eminence or more than 41% across the tibial plateau in the coronal plane.[36]
  - Calculation of the degree of correction[30]
    - o A line is created from the center of the femoral head through the apex of the lateral tibial eminence.
    - o A second line is drawn from the center of the talar dome through the same point on the tibia.
    - o The angle created by the intersection of these lines provides the degree of required correction and is translated laterally to the location of the most lateral cut on the proximal tibia.
    - o The height of the triangle created by the translated angle provides the required amount of correction of the osteotomy.
- o MRI
  - Evaluate soft tissue (ie, cartilage, meniscus, ligaments) and presence or absence of soft tissue fluid or joint effusion.
  - Unicompartmental bone edema can be indicator of chronic compartment overload.
  - Coronal or sagittal sequences can be used to assess meniscal volume
    - Caution should be used when evaluating meniscal injury following prior meniscal surgery. Most patients undergoing HTO have had previous meniscal surgery.
  - T2-weighted or short τ inversion recovery fluid sequences are used to evaluate cartilage or subchondral bone edema.
  - Gradient echo sequences are used to evaluate articular cartilage.
    - Note: The gradient echo sequence is unable to identify intrasubstance cartilage defects.
- o Computed tomography scans
  - Assist in assessing bone tunnel enlargement in cases of previous ACL reconstruction.

SURGICAL TECHNIQUE

- Positioning
  - o Patient is placed supine on the operating table with the nonoperative leg secured to the table.
  - o A high-thigh tourniquet is placed on the operative leg and a foot post is placed distal to the gastric bulge so that knee rests in full extension.

- Note: HTO has a tendency to increase posterior slope. This can be minimized by positioning the leg to ensure full extension during plate fixation.
- Note: A second foot post can be placed more proximally to allow positioning of the knee in 90° of flexion.
- HTO
  - The medial knee is marked for preparation for the meniscal transplant and HTO.
    - Note: The osteotomy is performed first. The meniscal slot is a stress riser on the tibial plateau, and if created first, the osteotomy could propagate into the slot and tibial plateau during opening of the osteotomy.
  - An anteromedial incision is made beginning midway between the tibial tubercle and the posteromedial border of the tibia. The incision is extended proximally to the mid-patella and distally to below the pes anserine.
  - The pes anserine is exposed. The sartorius fascia is incised in line with the gracilis tendon and the pes is mobilized posteriorly, exposing the medial collateral ligament (MCL) (**Fig. 1**)
  - The fascia along the medial border of the patella tendon is incised and the bursa just proximal of the tibial insertion of the patella tendon is opened.
  - The fascia posterior to the MCL is incised parallel to the MCL (**Fig. 2**). The popliteus muscle is released from the posteromedial tibia, always staying on bone with the dissection. After approximately 2 cm, the remaining posterior dissection can be performed bluntly until the fibular head can be palpated.
  - A posterior retractor is placed to protect the neurovascular bundle (**Fig. 3**).

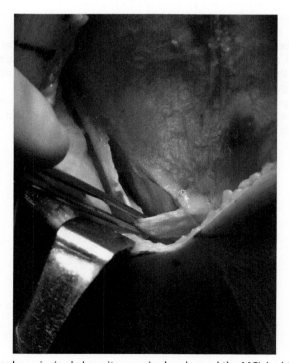

Fig. 1. The pes has been incised along its superior border and the MCL is visible underneath.

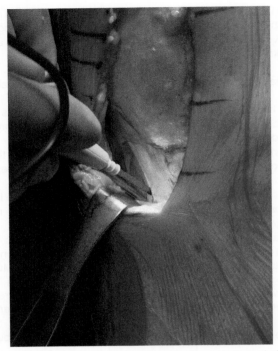

Fig. 2. The pes has been retracted posteriorly and the fascia is incised along the posterior border of the MCL.

- ○ Two guide pins are placed approximately parallel to the tibial slope distal to the tibial metaphyseal flare. The starting position is approximately at the level of the pes and the pins aim toward the proximal half of the fibular head (**Fig. 4**)
  - ■ It is important to maintain at least 1.5 cm of bone stock between the articular surface and the osteotomy site to prevent intraarticular fracture and to allow enough space for implant fixation.

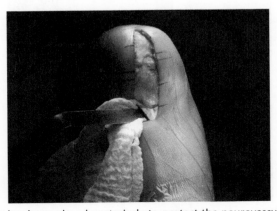

Fig. 3. A retractor has been placed posteriorly to protect the neurovascular bundle.

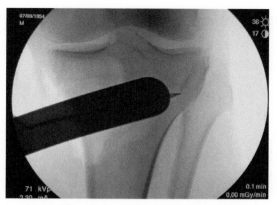

Fig. 4. A pin has been placed obliquely across the proximal tibia under fluoroscopic guidance.

- The superficial MCL is either cut at the level of the guide pin (**Fig. 5**), or the entire superficial MCL is mobilized and retracted posteriorly to expose the medial tibia.
  - Note: if the MCL is mobilized rather than cut, it has to be mobilized in its entirety distally to allow distraction of the osteotomy site.
- An oscillating saw is used to create the osteotomy (**Fig. 6**). Osteotomes are then used to advance the osteotomy along the medial, anterior, and posterior cortices.
  - It is imperative to use fluoroscopy to prevent damage to the lateral cortex and maintain at least 1 cm of a lateral bone hinge.
  - If the lateral cortex is fractured, a staple can be placed to prevent further propagation of the damage.
- A spreader device is used to slowly distract the medial cortex.
- Osteotomy tines are advanced into the osteotomy site to the amount of desired medial opening (**Fig. 7**).
- The osteotomy site is secured with a locking plate system (**Fig. 8**).
- Autologous bone graft and/or allograft can be used to pack the osteotomy site.

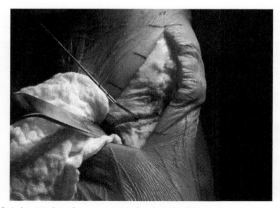

Fig. 5. The superficial MCL has been cut at the level of the pin.

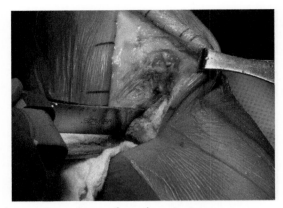

Fig. 6. An oscillating saw is used to perform the osteotomy.

- ○ A final fluoroscopic image is obtained to verify that the screws are of appropriate length, the osteotomy site is packed with bone graft, and the lateral cortex remains intact
- Meniscus transplantation
  - ○ A fresh-frozen nonirradiated meniscal allograft is preferred
  - ○ The size of the graft is determined preoperatively by[26]
    - ■ Meniscal width (medial-lateral dimension)
      - • Coronal distance from peak of medial tibial eminence to a line that is perpendicular to the joint line.
    - ■ Meniscal length (anteroposterior dimension)
      - • 80% of the sagittal length of the tibial plateau.
  - ○ The meniscus is prepared by placing a traction suture at the junction between the posterior horn and body. A bone bridge is created that connects anterior and posterior roots. There are several systems available, this article describes the bridge-in-slot technique (**Fig. 9**).
    - ■ Note: Although generally, medial meniscus allograft transplantation is performed with bone plugs rather than a bridge, the bridge technique is preferred with concomitant HTO, because with this technique meniscal fixation to the tibia is performed exclusively above the level of the osteotomy.

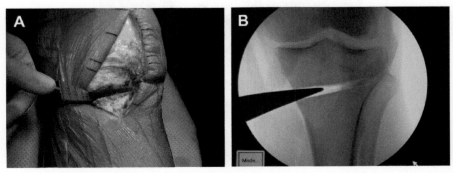

Fig. 7. The osteotomy is wedged open (*A*) under fluoroscopic control (*B*).

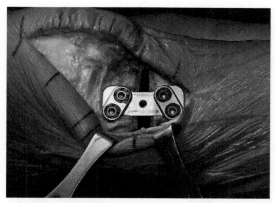

Fig. 8. The osteotomy has been secured with a locking plate.

- Standard anteromedial and anterolateral portals are established and diagnostic arthroscopy is performed.
- Several small perforations (pie-crusting) are made on the MCL to allow for increased medial compartment space.
- The medial meniscus is assessed, and any remaining medial meniscus is removed with an 11-blade scalpel and arthroscopic shaver, leaving a 1-mm rim of bleeding meniscal tissue.
- The integrity of the cartilage in the medial and lateral compartment is assessed. If there is a defect on the medial femoral condyle, this can be addressed with concomitant cartilage repair based on established algorithms.
- A long, flexible nitinol suture-passing pin and curved meniscal repair cannula is used to place a traction suture to exit the capsule at the posterior horn/body junction (**Fig. 10**).
- A slot is created in the tibial plateau, connecting anterior and posterior root attachment sites. First, overlying cartilage is debrided with electrocautery,

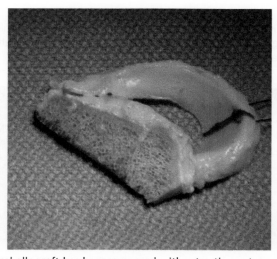

Fig. 9. The meniscal allograft has been prepared with a traction suture and bone bridge.

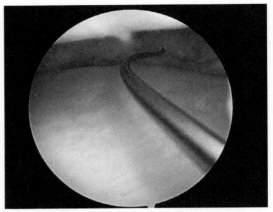

Fig. 10. A completion meniscectomy has been performed and a nitinol wire placed at the junction between the posterior horn and body.

then a trough is created with a burr, and finally a slot is created by using an 8-mm reamer deep to the trough and removing the bone in between. This can be performed arthroscopically or open (**Fig. 11**).

- Note: the slot will affect up to 25% of the ACL tibial footprint on its medial aspect.
- An accessory posteromedial incision is created, protecting the saphenous nerve.
- The prepared medial meniscal allograft is introduced into the medial compartment through the arthrotomy and pulled into position with the traction sutures at the posterior horn/body junction while pushing the bridge into the slot (**Fig. 12**).
- Once fully seated, the bridge is secured in the slot with an interference screw.
- The meniscal allograft is secured to the remnant meniscus and capsule with several vertical mattress sutures analogous to bucket-handle meniscus repair.

The wound is irrigated with normal saline, closed in layers, sterile dressings are applied, a cooling unit is incorporated into the dressing, and the patient is placed in a hinged knee brace locked in extension.

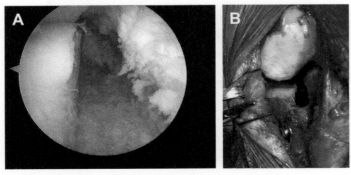

Fig. 11. The slot has been created arthroscopically (*A*) or open (*B*).

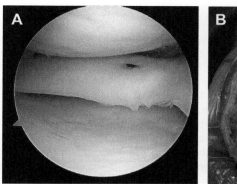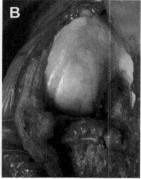

Fig. 12. The meniscus has been seated. Arthroscopic (*A*) or open (*B*) technique.

POSTOPERATIVE REHABILITATION

Following HTO with concomitant medial MAT with or without osteochondral allograft transplant, a standard rehabilitation protocol is implemented by the senior author (**Table 2**).

Table 2
Standard rehabilitation protocol following high tibial osteotomy and concomitant medial meniscal allograft transplant

Phase	Weight-Bearing Status	Brace	Range of Motion	Exercises
Phase 1 0–2 wk	Touch-down weight bearing	Locked in full extension at all times. May be removed for hygiene and home exercises only.	Gentle passive 0°–60°	Heel slides, quad sets, patellar mobs, straight leg raise, calf pumps
Phase 2 2–6 wk	Touch-down weight bearing	Locked in full extension for ambulation only. Can discard for sleeping.	0–90	Add side-lying hip and core, straight leg raises, advance quad set and gentle stretching
Phase 3 7–12 wk	Full	None	Full	Add heel raises, gait normalization, eccentric quadriceps and hamstrings Squat/leg press 0°-90° only, proprioception/balance exercises Begin stationary bike
Phase 4 12–24 wk	Full	None	Full	Progress Phase 3 exercises and functional activities: walking lunges, plants, bridges, swiss ball, half-bosu exercises Advance core/gluteals and balance
Phase 5 6–9 mo	Full	None	Full	Advance all activity w/o impact (ie, running, jumping, pivoting, sports) until cleared by physician

OUTCOMES

Following HTO, patients demonstrate improvements in patient-reported outcome measures, high patient satisfaction, and procedural survivorship.[8–11] Although patients demonstrate improvements in functional or clinical outcomes, these metrics may exhibit a ceiling effect and may not capture the true improvement in younger, active patients. Following HTO, 85% to 87% of patients were able to return to sport and 85% of patients were able to return to work.[6,37] Despite a high rate of return to sport and work, only 79% and 66% of patients were able to return to their preoperative level of function.[37] A known complication in 12% to 35% cases of HTO is a lateral hinge fracture that occurs during distraction of the medial cortex.[38] However, there was no significant difference in radiographic measurements (ie, hip-knee-ankle angle, femorotibial angle, medial proximal tibial angle, and posterior tibial slope angle), functional outcomes, complications, or correction loss in patients with a lateral hinge fracture.[39] It is important to note that performing a HTO in patients with discoid lateral meniscus may accelerate osteoarthritis in the lateral compartment.[40]

Concomitant HTO and ACL reconstruction has been described as a salvage procedure in patients with chronic ACL deficiency.[41] Regardless of surgical intervention, ACL deficiency accelerates cartilage loss on the medial femoral condyle[42] as well as medial meniscal lesions.[43] Meniscal damage following ACL deficiency further compounds the damage caused by varus malalignment.[44] Young, active patients undergoing simultaneous HTO and ACL reconstruction demonstrated restoration of anterior stability, alleviation of medial compartment osteoarthritis, improvement in functional outcome metrics, as well as a high rate of return to sport.[45]

Although MAT is an efficacious treatment modality to ameliorate symptoms in meniscus-deficient knees, it has been shown that concomitant ligament instability, axis malalignment, or advanced cartilage defects results in inferior outcomes.[46–49] Although MAT may be most efficacious in a young, active individual with isolated meniscal deficiency, at least one concomitant procedure is performed in more than half of MATs.[50] In a systematic review, Lee and colleagues[51] demonstrated no statistical difference in patient-reported outcome measures between isolated MAT and MAT with concomitant procedures. Following MAT, 74% of patients were able to return to sport with only 49% of patients being able to return to their previous level of activity.[52] This case series is of particular interest due the proportion of concomitant high tibial osteotomies (29%) included in its analysis. However, a subgroup analysis of HTO with concomitant MAT was not performed. Furthermore, Verdonk and colleagues[20] demonstrated in a series of 13 patients that HTO with concomitant medial meniscal transplant resulted in an improvement in pain and function as well as cumulative survival rate and duration of 83.3% and 13.0 years, respectively. Concomitant HTO may improve outcomes following MAT by relieving pressure in the medial compartment. However, clinical outcomes following concomitant HTO and MAT is lacking and future investigations are needed to elucidate outcomes following these concomitant procedures.

Patients undergoing MAT with concomitant chondral lesions may also be treated with cartilage restoration procedures, such as autologous chondrocyte implantation, microfracture, or osteochondral graft fixation. Saltzman and colleagues[53] demonstrate that this population of patients have equivalent functional outcomes as those patients with no chondral lesions. HTO with cartilage restoration procedures have also been shown to provide reliable improvements in pain relief and functional outcome scores in patients with focal chondral defects.[15] The most commonly performed cartilage restoration procedures included microfracture as well as autologous chondrocyte transfer; however, their efficacy is inconclusive.[54,55] HTO can be augmented with platelet-rich plasma (PRP) or mesenchymal stem cells (MSCs) to improve cartilage healing. In a prospective analysis, Koh and colleagues[56] demonstrated that HTO with MSC augmentation improved cartilage healing more than PRP as identified through second-look arthroscopy. Furthermore, patients with MSC augmentation demonstrated improvements in patient-reported outcome measures. However, these findings must be interpreted with caution as patients were not blinded to their treatment group and improvements may be a byproduct of a placebo effect. Clinical outcomes and regeneration of cartilage following concomitant HTO and cartilage procedures is lacking; therefore, future investigations are needed to establish outcomes following HTO with cartilage restoration procedures.

SUMMARY

In patients with medial meniscal deficiency and varus malalignment, there are several available treatment options such as injections, meniscal transplant, or osteotomy. HTO with concomitant medial MAT is an appropriate treatment option for younger, active patients who wish to continue an active lifestyle. To optimize patient outcomes, it is imperative that patients meet selection criteria. Furthermore, preoperative consultation is important in management of expectations, especially in younger patients who are more motivated and may have higher expectations of their osteotomy.[57,58] Outcomes following HTO with concomitant medial MAT needs to be better defined. However, achieving a sufficient sample size may be difficult given the rarity of this procedure.

REFERENCES

1. Aujla RS, Esler CN. Total knee arthroplasty for osteoarthritis in patients less than fifty-five years of age: a systematic review. J Arthroplasty 2017;32(8):2598–603.e1.
2. Witjes S, van Geenen RC, Koenraadt KL, et al. Expectations of younger patients concerning activities after knee arthroplasty: are we asking the right questions? Qual Life Res 2017;26(2):403–17.
3. Coventry MB. Osteotomy of the upper portion of the tibia for degenerative arthritis of the knee. A preliminary report. J Bone Joint Surg Am 1965;47:984–90.
4. Smith JO, Wilson AJ, Thomas NP. Osteotomy around the knee: evolution, principles and results. Knee Surg Sports Traumatol Arthrosc 2013;21(1):3–22.
5. Wright JM, Crockett HC, Slawski DP, et al. High tibial osteotomy. J Am Acad Orthop Surg 2005;13(4):279–89.
6. Hoorntje A, Witjes S, Kuijer P, et al. High rates of return to sports activities and work after osteotomies around the knee: a systematic review and meta-analysis. Sports Med 2017;47(11):2219–44.
7. Konopka JF, Gomoll AH, Thornhill TS, et al. The cost-effectiveness of surgical treatment of medial unicompartmental knee osteoarthritis in younger patients: a computer model-based evaluation. J Bone Joint Surg Am 2015;97(10):807–17.
8. Bode G, von Heyden J, Pestka J, et al. Prospective 5-year survival rate data following open-wedge valgus high tibial osteotomy. Knee Surg Sports Traumatol Arthrosc 2015;23(7):1949–55.
9. Hui C, Salmon LJ, Kok A, et al. Long-term survival of high tibial osteotomy for medial compartment osteoarthritis of the knee. Am J Sports Med 2011;39(1):64–70.
10. Niemeyer P, Schmal H, Hauschild O, et al. Open-wedge osteotomy using an internal plate fixator in patients with medial-compartment gonarthritis and varus malalignment: 3-year results with regard to preoperative arthroscopic and radiographic findings. Arthroscopy 2010;26(12):1607–16.

11. Schallberger A, Jacobi M, Wahl P, et al. High tibial valgus osteotomy in unicompartmental medial osteoarthritis of the knee: a retrospective follow-up study over 13-21 years. Knee Surg Sports Traumatol Arthrosc 2011;19(1):122–7.
12. Cameron JI, McCauley JC, Kermanshahi AY, et al. Lateral opening-wedge distal femoral osteotomy: pain relief, functional improvement, and survivorship at 5 years. Clin Orthop Relat Res 2015;473(6):2009–15.
13. Niinimaki TT, Eskelinen A, Ohtonen P, et al. Incidence of osteotomies around the knee for the treatment of knee osteoarthritis: a 22-year population-based study. Int Orthop 2012;36(7):1399–402.
14. Brinkman JM, Lobenhoffer P, Agneskirchner JD, et al. Osteotomies around the knee: patient selection, stability of fixation and bone healing in high tibial osteotomies. J Bone Joint Surg Br 2008;90(12):1548–57.
15. Kahlenberg CA, Nwachukwu BU, Hamid KS, et al. Analysis of outcomes for high tibial osteotomies performed with cartilage restoration techniques. Arthroscopy 2017;33(2):486–92.
16. Verdonk PC, Demurie A, Almqvist KF, et al. Transplantation of viable meniscal allograft. Surgical technique. J Bone Joint Surg Am 2006;88(Suppl 1 Pt 1):109–18.
17. Vundelinckx B, Bellemans J, Vanlauwe J. Arthroscopically assisted meniscal allograft transplantation in the knee: a medium-term subjective, clinical, and radiographical outcome evaluation. Am J Sports Med 2010;38(11):2240–7.
18. van Arkel ER, de Boer HH. Survival analysis of human meniscal transplantations. J Bone Joint Surg Br 2002;84(2):227–31.
19. van der Wal RJ, Thomassen BJ, van Arkel ER. Long-term clinical outcome of open meniscal allograft transplantation. Am J Sports Med 2009;37(11):2134–9.
20. Verdonk PC, Demurie A, Almqvist KF, et al. Transplantation of viable meniscal allograft. Survivorship analysis and clinical outcome of one hundred cases. J Bone Joint Surg Am 2005;87(4):715–24.
21. Yoon KH, Lee SH, Park SY, et al. Meniscus allograft transplantation: a comparison of medial and lateral procedures. Am J Sports Med 2014;42(1):200–7.
22. Vundelinckx B, Vanlauwe J, Bellemans J. Long-term subjective, clinical, and radiographic outcome evaluation of meniscal allograft transplantation in the knee. Am J Sports Med 2014;42(7):1592–9.
23. Bin SI, Nha KW, Cheong JY, et al. Midterm and long-term results of medial versus lateral meniscal allograft transplantation: a meta-analysis. Am J Sports Med 2018; 46(5):1243–50.
24. Verdonk PC, Verstraete KL, Almqvist KF, et al. Meniscal allograft transplantation: long-term clinical results with radiological and magnetic resonance imaging correlations. Knee Surg Sports Traumatol Arthrosc 2006;14(8):694–706.
25. Rossi R, Bonasia DE, Amendola A. The role of high tibial osteotomy in the varus knee. J Am Acad Orthop Surg 2011;19(10):590–9.
26. LaPrade RF, Oro FB, Ziegler CG, et al. Patellar height and tibial slope after opening-wedge proximal tibial osteotomy: a prospective study. Am J Sports Med 2010;38(1):160–70.
27. Jackman T, LaPrade RF, Pontinen T, et al. Intraobserver and interobserver reliability of the kneeling technique of stress radiography for the evaluation of posterior knee laxity. Am J Sports Med 2008;36(8):1571–6.
28. Kolb W, Guhlmann H, Windisch C, et al. Opening-wedge high tibial osteotomy with a locked low-profile plate. J Bone Joint Surg Am 2009;91(11):2581–8.
29. Kolb W, Guhlmann H, Windisch C, et al. Opening-wedge high tibial osteotomy with a locked low-profile plate: surgical technique. J Bone Joint Surg Am 2010; 92(Suppl 1 Pt 2):197–207.

30. Chahla J, Dean CS, Mitchell JJ, et al. Medial opening wedge proximal tibial osteotomy. Arthrosc Tech 2016;5(4):e919–28.

31. Han JH, Yang JH, Bhandare NN, et al. Total knee arthroplasty after failed high tibial osteotomy: a systematic review of open versus closed wedge osteotomy. Knee Surg Sports Traumatol Arthrosc 2016;24(8):2567–77.

32. Bastos Filho R, Magnussen RA, Duthon V, et al. Total knee arthroplasty after high tibial osteotomy: a comparison of opening and closing wedge osteotomy. Int Orthop 2013;37(3):427–31.

33. Nerhus TK, Ekeland A, Solberg G, et al. No difference in time-dependent improvement in functional outcome following closing wedge versus opening wedge high tibial osteotomy: a randomised controlled trial with two-year follow-up. Bone Joint J 2017;99-B(9):1157–66.

34. Duivenvoorden T, van Diggele P, Reijman M, et al. Adverse events and survival after closing- and opening-wedge high tibial osteotomy: a comparative study of 412 patients. Knee Surg Sports Traumatol Arthrosc 2017;25(3):895–901.

35. Clarke JV, Nunn T. The reproducibility and repeatability of varus stress radiographs in the assessment of isolated fibular collateral ligament and grade-III posterolateral knee injuries. J Bone Joint Surg Am 2009;91(2):485 [author reply: 485–6].

36. Laprade RF, Spiridonov SI, Nystrom LM, et al. Prospective outcomes of young and middle-aged adults with medial compartment osteoarthritis treated with a proximal tibial opening wedge osteotomy. Arthroscopy 2012;28(3):354–64.

37. Ekhtiari S, Haldane CE, de Sa D, et al. Return to work and sport following high tibial osteotomy: a systematic review. J Bone Joint Surg Am 2016;98(18):1568–77.

38. Lee OS, Lee YS. Diagnostic value of computed tomography and risk factors for lateral hinge fracture in the open wedge high tibial osteotomy. Arthroscopy 2018;34(4):1032–43.

39. Kim KI, Kim GB, Kim HJ, et al. Extra-articular lateral hinge fracture does not affect the outcomes in medial open-wedge high tibial osteotomy using a locked plate system. Arthroscopy 2018;34(12):3246–55.

40. Prakash J, Song EK, Lim HA, et al. High tibial osteotomy accelerates lateral compartment osteoarthritis in discoid meniscus patients. Knee Surg Sports Traumatol Arthrosc 2018;26(6):1845–50.

41. O'Neill DF, James SL. Valgus osteotomy with anterior cruciate ligament laxity. Clin Orthop Relat Res 1992;278:153–9.

42. Potter HG, Jain SK, Ma Y, et al. Cartilage injury after acute, isolated anterior cruciate ligament tear: immediate and longitudinal effect with clinical/MRI follow-up. Am J Sports Med 2012;40(2):276–85.

43. Guenther ZD, Swami V, Dhillon SS, et al. Meniscal injury after adolescent anterior cruciate ligament injury: how long are patients at risk? Clin Orthop Relat Res 2014;472(3):990–7.

44. Bonasia DE, Dettoni F, Sito G, et al. Medial opening wedge high tibial osteotomy for medial compartment overload/arthritis in the varus knee: prognostic factors. Am J Sports Med 2014;42(3):690–8.

45. Li Y, Zhang H, Zhang J, et al. Clinical outcome of simultaneous high tibial osteotomy and anterior cruciate ligament reconstruction for medial compartment osteoarthritis in young patients with anterior cruciate ligament-deficient knees: a systematic review. Arthroscopy 2015;31(3):507–19.

46. Cameron JC, Saha S. Meniscal allograft transplantation for unicompartmental arthritis of the knee. Clin Orthop Relat Res 1997;337:164–71.

47. Getgood A, Gelber J, Gortz S, et al. Combined osteochondral allograft and meniscal allograft transplantation: a survivorship analysis. Knee Surg Sports Traumatol Arthrosc 2015;23(4):946–53.

48. Harris JD, Cavo M, Brophy R, et al. Biological knee reconstruction: a systematic review of combined meniscal allograft transplantation and cartilage repair or restoration. Arthroscopy 2011;27(3):409–18.

49. Kempshall PJ, Parkinson B, Thomas M, et al. Outcome of meniscal allograft transplantation related to articular cartilage status: advanced chondral damage should not be a contraindication. Knee Surg Sports Traumatol Arthrosc 2015; 23(1):280–9.

50. Rosso F, Bisicchia S, Bonasia DE, et al. Meniscal allograft transplantation: a systematic review. Am J Sports Med 2015;43(4):998–1007.

51. Lee BS, Kim HJ, Lee CR, et al. Clinical outcomes of meniscal allograft transplantation with or without other procedures: a systematic review and meta-analysis. Am J Sports Med 2018;46(12):3047–56.

52. Zaffagnini S, Grassi A, Marcheggiani Muccioli GM, et al. Is sport activity possible after arthroscopic meniscal allograft transplantation? midterm results in active patients. Am J Sports Med 2016;44(3):625–32.

53. Saltzman BM, Meyer MA, Leroux TS, et al. The influence of full-thickness chondral defects on outcomes following meniscal allograft transplantation: a comparative study. Arthroscopy 2018;34(2):519–29.

54. Safran MR, Seiber K. The evidence for surgical repair of articular cartilage in the knee. J Am Acad Orthop Surg 2010;18(5):259–66.

55. Lee OS, Ahn S, Ahn JH, et al. Effectiveness of concurrent procedures during high tibial osteotomy for medial compartment osteoarthritis: a systematic review and meta-analysis. Arch Orthop Trauma Surg 2018;138(2):227–36.

56. Koh YG, Kwon OR, Kim YS, et al. Comparative outcomes of open-wedge high tibial osteotomy with platelet-rich plasma alone or in combination with mesenchymal stem cell treatment: a prospective study. Arthroscopy 2014;30(11): 1453–60.

57. Bonnin MP, Laurent JR, Zadegan F, et al. Can patients really participate in sport after high tibial osteotomy? Knee Surg Sports Traumatol Arthrosc 2013;21(1): 64–73.

58. Grunwald L, Angele P, Schroter S, et al. Patients' expectations of osteotomies around the knee are high regarding activities of daily living. Knee Surg Sports Traumatol Arthrosc 2018. [Epub ahead of print].

High Tibial Osteotomy and Anterior Cruciate Ligament Reconstruction/Revision

Antonino Cantivalli, MD[a], Federica Rosso, MD[b],*,
Davide Edoardo Bonasia, MD[b], Roberto Rossi, MD[a,b]

KEYWORDS

- High tibial osteotomy • ACL reconstruction • ACL reconstruction revision
- Knee instability • Varus alignment

KEY POINTS

- High tibial osteotomy (HTO) is a procedure commonly used to treat medial early osteoarthritis (OA) in young and active patients.
- Combined HTO and anterior cruciate ligament reconstruction (ACL-R) is indicated in patients with medial OA (Ahlbäck I-III) and varus alignment (primary, double, or triple varus) associated with ACL tear with symptomatic anteroposterior instability, failed ACL-R, or increased posterior tibial slope (PTS).
- A PTS greater than 12° is a risk factor for ACL-R failure and should be modified.
- There are different surgical techniques to perform a concomitant HTO and ACL-R. Opening wedge and closing wedge HTO are the most commonly performed, but there is no evidence supporting the superiority of one procedure over the others. For ACL-R, soft tissue autograft or allograft is commonly used in association with anatomic reconstruction.
- There are few studies on combined HTO and ACL-R with short follow-up and few patients. However, most of these studies reported good outcomes, with complication rates similar to isolated or staged ACL-R.

INTRODUCTION

High tibial osteotomy (HTO) is generally performed to treat young active patients with medial tibiofemoral osteoarthrosis (OA) and varus deformity.[1–3] There are many different techniques to perform an HTO, such as closing wedge osteotomy (CWHTO), opening wedge osteotomy (OWHTO), dome osteotomy, progressive callus

Disclosure Statement: R. Rossi is a teaching consultant for Zimmer Biomet, Depuy Mitek, Medacta, Lima Corporate, and Smith and Nephew. The other authors certify that they have no commercial associations that might pose a conflict of interest in connection with the submitted article.
[a] University of Study of Turin, Via Po 8, Turin 10100, Italy; [b] Department of Orthopedics and Traumatology, AO Ordine Mauriziano, Largo Turati 62, Turin 10128, Italy
* Corresponding author.
E-mail address: federica.rosso@yahoo.it

Clin Sports Med 38 (2019) 417–433
https://doi.org/10.1016/j.csm.2019.02.008
0278-5919/19/© 2019 Elsevier Inc. All rights reserved.

sportsmed.theclinics.com

distraction, and "en chevron" osteotomy.[4] However, OWHTO and CTHTO are the most commonly performed, but there is no evidence supporting the superiority of 1 procedure over the others.[5] In the presence of medial OA and chronic anterior cruciate ligament (ACL) deficiency, patients may develop cartilage wear of the posteromedial tibial plateau with worsening of the varus deformity and progressive slackening of the lateral and posterolateral ligamentous structures, with lateral joint opening.[6–8] This concept has been previously described as primary, double, and triple varus by Noyes and colleagues.[6] Primary varus refers to tibiofemoral osseous alignment and geometry of the knee, including the varus alignment occurring after medial meniscectomy and damage to the medial articular cartilage.[9] "Double varus" refers to the presence of varus alignment due to tibiofemoral osseous alignment associated with lateral joint space opening due to lateral soft tissue slackening. These patients normally present a varus thrust when ambulating.[6] When chronic tensile forces continue to stress the posterolateral ligament structures, a varus recurvatum is added, resulting in the so-called triple varus.[6,8] In these cases, the varus deformity is due to tibiofemoral varus alignment, lateral joint space opening, and increased external tibial rotation and hyperextension, with an abnormal varus recurvatum position.[6] Triple varus cases are most commonly a consequence of chronic posterior cruciate ligament and posterolateral corner deficiency. Some investigators demonstrated that, in patients with double or triple varus, there are different gait abnormalities, such as decreased flexion moment, increased external adduction moment, increased external knee extension moment, and increased hyperextension during stance phase.[10,11] Furthermore, posterior tibial slope (PTS) also plays an important role in the ACL-deficient varus knees. Different investigators demonstrated that, in the ACL-deficient knee, anterior tibial translation can be reduced by decreasing the PTS[12] to normal values (normal value in medial plateau 9°–11°, in lateral plateau 6°–8°).[13–16] Furthermore, decreasing the PTS helps in reducing the tension forces on ACL, with a consequent reduced risk of rerupture of the graft.[13,15–18] Conversely, an increased PTS increases the forces on ACL with consequently increased risk for graft rupture.[13,15,16] PTS may be modified during OWHTO, depending on the gap height. Noyes and colleagues[19] demonstrated that, in order not to change the PTS in OWHTO, the anterior gap height should be half of the posteromedial one. Conversely, if the anterior gap is bigger than the posterior gap, PTS will be increased. For these reasons, despite that PTS may be changed with either CWHTO or OWHTO, it can be fine-tuned during OWHTO. If a toothed plate is used, in particular, the PTS can be easily increased or decreased depending on plate positioning, according to trigonometric rules. However, PTS can also be easily corrected and fine-tuned using locking plates during OWHTO.[20] Some investigators demonstrated that for each increase of 1 mm in the anterior gap compared with the posterior one, the PTS increases 2°.[19] For all these reasons, in patients with important varus alignment and medial OA associated with ACL failure due to increased PTS, the coronal and sagittal alignment may be corrected with an HTO performed in association with the ACL reconstruction (ACL-R)/revision.[21]

The aim of this article is to summarize the most recent literature about the indication, preoperative planning, surgical technique, and outcomes of HTO performed in association with ACL-R/revision.

INDICATIONS

HTO and ACL-R/revision may be performed in a "1-stage" or in a "2-stage" procedure. However, in both cases, correct patient selection is mandatory to achieve a good outcome.[1,6,9,22,23]

The "1-stage" procedure, defined as concomitant HTO and ACL-R/revision, is indicated in young patients with (1) Medial-compartment OA (Ahlbäck I-III) associated with varus malalignment and ACL tear with symptomatic anteroposterior (AP) instability[24]; (2) Medial-compartment OA (Ahlbäck I-III) associated with varus malalignment and failed ACL-[21,24]; (3) Failed ACL-R due to increased PTS[21]; (4) Double or triple varus and ACL tear with symptomatic AP instability[24]; (5) Varus malalignment associated with ACL tear and chondral or meniscal injuries requiring cartilage repair or meniscal transplant.[25] These indications and contraindications are summarized in **Table 1**.

Isolated HTO with possible delayed ACL-R/revision ("2-stage" procedure) is mostly indicated in older patients with (1) Chronic ACL deficiency (with no to minimal subjective AP instability) associated with double or triple varus; (2) Chronic ACL deficiency (with no to minimal subjective AP instability) associated with varus malalignment and symptomatic medial-compartment OA; (3) Chronic ACL deficiency (with no to minimal subjective AP instability) associated with double or triple varus and symptomatic medial-compartment OA.[15] These indications are summarized in **Table 1**. As previously described for double or triple varus, if posterolateral structures are lax and not completed disrupted, HTO alone tends to stabilize the knee and can avoid ligament reconstruction, especially when the major symptom is pain and not instability.[26] Ranawat and colleagues[27] confirmed that isolated HTO in the ACL-deficient knee improves

Table 1
Indication and contraindication for high tibial osteotomy and combined high tibial osteotomy and anterior cruciate ligament reconstruction

Indication for Combined HTO + ACLR vs Isolated HTO	
Combined HTO + ACL-R (One-Stage)	**Isolated HTO + Delayed ACL-R (Two-Stage)**
Medial OA (Ahlbäck grades 1–3) + varus malalignment + ACL lesion (AP instability)	Chronic ACL deficiency + double or triple varus
Medial OA (Ahlbäck grades 1–3) + varus malalignment + Failed ACL-R Increased PTS that led to ACL-R failure	Chronic ACL deficiency + varus alignment + medial OA
ACL tear + Double or triple varus Varus malalignment + ACL tear + chondral or meniscal injuries	Chronic ACL deficiency + double or triple varus + medial OA
Contraindications for HTO	
Severe articular damage of medial compartment (Ahlbäck grade III or higher)	
Tricompartmental arthrosis	
Patellofemoral arthrosis	
Decreased ROM <120° or flexion contracture >5°	
Age >65°	
BMI >30 (relative contraindication)	
Inflammatory disease	
Severe osteoporosis	

knee kinematics and tibiofemoral alignment by reducing PTS (in particular, an average PTS reduction of 7.1° for CWHTO and 5.1° for OWHTO), reducing lateral joint opening and decreasing the anterior tibial translation during Lachman test or anterior drawer test. On the other hand, severe articular damage (Ahlbäck grade III or higher),[1] advanced age (>65 years),[28] tricompartmental arthritis,[29] inflammatory disease,[20] severe osteoporosis, and decreased range of motion (ROM; <120° and flexion contracture >5°)[23] are generally considered contraindication for HTO alone or combined with ACL-R (see **Table 1**). The importance of body mass index (BMI) is controversial, but recent literature agrees that the ideal BMI to perform an HTO alone or in combination to ACL-R is between 25 and 27.5 kg/m². [23]

PREOPERATIVE PLANNING

A careful preoperative evaluation is mandatory. First, a complete radiographic evaluation, including AP and lateral weight-bearing long-leg views, as well as Merchant view at 30° of flexion and Rosenberg view at 45° of flexion, should be performed.[1] MRI is necessary to evaluate any other bony or soft tissue pathologic conditions (meniscal tears, osteonecrosis, osteochondral defects, ligamentous tears, and so forth), to identify subchondral edema or other signs of compartment overload and to assess the degree of medial compartment cartilage degeneration. Clinical evaluation, including gait, is also mandatory. Patients may demonstrate a varus thrust[6,30] in particular due to posterolateral soft tissue slackening.[31,32]

Preoperative planning is normally performed according to the method described by Dugdale and colleagues.[9] In most of the cases, a slight overcorrection, corresponding to about 62.5% of the tibial plate, is desired.[33] However, in young, active patients, or if a concomitant surgery, such as cartilage procedure or meniscal transplant, is performed, a neutral alignment (50% of the tibial plateau) should be achieved.[34]

If an OWHTO is planned, 1 line is drawn from lateral tibial spine (62.5% point on tibial plateau) to the center of the femoral head (line a), and another line is drawn from this point to the center of the ankle joint (line b). The angle between the 2 lines represents the correction angle (alpha). The osteotomy line is drawn on the proximal tibia from medial (4 cm below the joint line) to lateral (tip of the fibular head), and it is transferred to both the rays of the alfa angle. The distance between these segments (line bc) is equivalent to the toothed plate or the amount of medial opening required to obtain the planned correction. **Fig. 1** shows the planning. Surgical planning for CWHTO is similar. The alfa angle is calculated as described for OWHTO, but the osteotomy entails 2 cuts. The proximal cut is usually horizontal and 2 to 2.5 cm distal to the joint line, whereas the distal cut is performed with the planned angulation to create the right correction angle.[1] As a general rule, in CWHTO, 1 mm of bone removal corresponds to 1° of correction.[35] In the sagittal plane, the PTS should be evaluated, most of all, in cases of ACL-R failure,[1] and, if it is increased, it should be modified to reduce tension on the reconstructed ACL[15] and, consequently, the risk of rerupture.[36] Considering the triangular shape of the tibia, as described by Noyes and colleagues[19] during OWHTO, the anterior gap should be half of the posterior one to maintain PTS. If the plate is placed too anteriorly, the PTS will increase as previously described.[6,20]As described by Rodner and colleagues,[37] an anteromedial (AM) plate in particular increases the slope on average by 5.5°, whereas Marti and colleagues[38] reported about an average increase in PTS of 2.7° for every 10° of valgus correction with OWHTO. Last, the patellar height also should be carefully evaluated in the preoperative planning using the Insall-Salvati, Blackburne-Peel, or Caton-Dechamps index,[39] because there is a potential risk to generate a patella baja after an OWHTO. For this reason, some

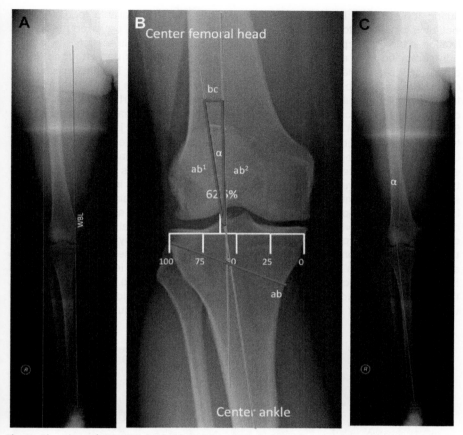

Fig. 1. Planning of OWHTO (right leg). (*A*) Long-leg view. The weight-bearing line is drawn from the center of the femoral head to the center of the ankle. In this image, the knee has a varus alignment. (*B*) OWHTO is planned with a line from the center of femoral head to the 62.5% tibial plateau (from medial to lateral, a line) and another line from the center of the ankle to the same point of tibial plateau (b line). The angle between the 2 lines (alpha) is the correction angle. The osteotomy line (ab) is performed from medial (4 cm under the joint line) to lateral (1 cm below the joint line). The length of ab line is transferred on both lines passing from 62.5% of the tibial plateau, and according to trigonometric rules, bc is equal to the opening needed. (*C*). Representation of the planning on the long-leg view.

investigators suggested performing a biplanar osteotomy (including the tibial tubercle) if the planned osteotomy is larger than 1 cm, to avoid patella baja.[1,20,23]

If a concomitant ACL-R/revision is planned, although it is possible to use bone block autograft or allograft (ie, bone-patellar tendon-bone or Achilles tendon), it may be better to use soft tissue autograft (ie, hamstring) or allograft (ie, tibialis anterior) to overcome the possible complication due to graft tunnel mismatch.[15]

SURGICAL TECHNIQUE

In most cases, if a combined ACL-R/revision and HTO is planned, an OWHTO is normally preferred by the investigators,[1] mostly because the slope may be corrected during the surgery. There are different fixation methods available for OWHTO,[23] including locking or toothed plate (Puddu plate).[4] The authors' preferred method for fixation is the Puddu plate, so this technique is described in this section.

In combined HTO and ACL-R/revision, the osteotomy must be performed first[40]; otherwise the graft may be damaged during the tibial bone cut. The patient is supine, on a radiolucent table with a tourniquet and a lateral post at the proximal thigh.[41] Patient positioning should allow for knee hyperflexion for transportal inside-out femoral drilling. The surgery can be performed in either general or spinal anesthesia. A 7- to 8-cm vertical incision is performed medially, 1 cm distal to the joint line, halfway between the medial tubercle and the posteromedial tibial cortex, as in a standard OWHTO. If an autologous hamstring graft is used, the sartorial fascia is incised to expose the gracilis tendon proximally and the semitendinosus tendon distally, and the tendons are harvested in a standard manner. Arthroscopy is performed through standard AM and anterolateral portals. A complete knee evaluation is performed, including menisci and cartilage. The ACL stump is removed, and the intercondylar notch is carefully debrided at the medial wall of the lateral femoral condyle. Sometimes osteophytes may be present in the intercondylar notch, and they need to be removed to avoid roof impingement with the ACL graft. ACL femoral tunnel should be placed in an anatomic position. The authors' preferred technique is the inside-out transportal femoral drilling, especially in ACL primary reconstruction (**Fig. 2**).[15] In ACL-R revision, the technique to perform the femoral tunnel may change considering the position of the previous tunnels (ie, "over the top" or outside-in technique).[42] If a transportal

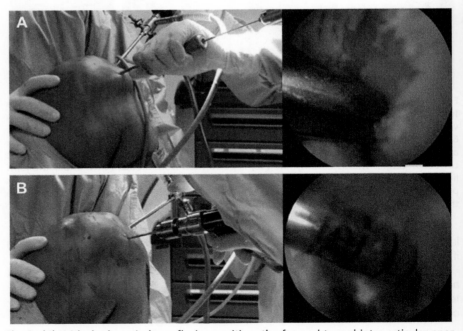

Fig. 2. (*A*) With the knee in hyperflexion position, the femoral tunnel intra-articular aperture is determined (usually the AM bundle or halfway between the AM and PL bundles): on the right is reported the arthroscopic view. (*B*) A cannulated reamer is used to create a full tunnel over the guidewire with the inside-out technique: arthroscopic view on the right. PL, posterolateral.

femoral tunnel is performed, a femoral offset guide may be used to place a guidewire at the desired position for the femoral tunnel (see **Fig. 2**A). If an extracortical suspension technique is preferred, a dedicated cannulated reamer is used to create a full tunnel over the guidewire (see **Fig** 2B). After the tunnel is measured, a half tunnel of the desired length is created with the cannulated reamer of the same size of the graft diameter. A shuttle suture is positioned in the femoral tunnel, exiting from the lateral thigh and the AM portal.[15] At this point, the osteotomy is performed, after superficial medial collateral ligament is partially released.[23] A guidewire is positioned under radiographic guidance from medial to lateral and from distal to proximal, from 4 cm below the medial joint line toward the tip of fibular head (1 cm below the lateral joint line). A 3-cm-wide, thin oscillating saw and thin osteotomes are used to cut the medial, anterior, and posteromedial cortex, being careful not to break the lateral hinge (**Fig. 3**). The osteotomy should be parallel to the tibial slope (10° of AP inclination). The osteotome should be advanced within 1 cm from the lateral tibial cortex. This distance should be less than the distance between the lateral joint line and the osteotomy to avoid intra-articular migration of the osteotomy.[43] The osteotomy is gradually opened using piled osteotomes, being careful not to break the lateral cortex. Once the osteotomy site has been partially opened, graduated wedges can be placed (**Fig. 4**). Under fluoroscopy control, a long alignment rod is placed from the center of the femoral head to the center of the ankle to check the mechanical axis of the knee. Once the desired osteotomy opening and alignment correction are achieved, the corresponding plate is positioned at the osteotomy site, leaving the wedges. In combined HTO and ACL-R, the plate is generally positioned in a more posterior position compared with isolated HTO to decrease the tibial slope, to reduce the tension forces on the ACL, and to leave more space on the anteromedial tibia for tibial tunnel drilling.[15]

For osteotomies larger than 10 mm, a bone graft is necessary (iliac crest autograft, allograft, or bone substitutes) to reduce the risk of nonunion.[4,15,20] The plate is fixed with all the screws except for the proximal anterior cancellous screw, which will be inserted after the tibial tunnel drilling.[15]

Under arthroscopic evaluation, a guidewire is positioned at the tibial ACL footprint using dedicated instrumentation. The tibial aperture of the tunnel should be right

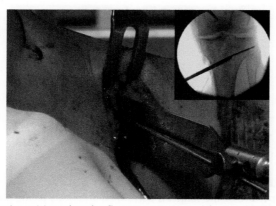

Fig. 3. A guidewire is positioned under fluoroscopic control from medial to lateral and from distal to proximal, 4 cm under the joint line medially and 1 cm laterally. The osteotomy is created distally to the guidewire in order to avoid proximal migration of the osteotomy toward the articulation. At the beginning, a thin oscillating saw is used; then a graduated osteotome is used to create the osteotomy.

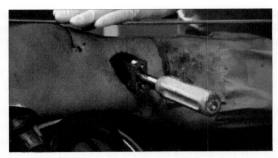

Fig. 4. The osteotomy is gradually opened using multiple and progressive osteotomes and dedicated instrumentation 8 as in the figure), being careful not to break the lateral cortex.

anterior to the plate into the proximal tibial fragment (**Fig. 5**). The guidewire is over-drilled with a cannulated reamer of the same size of the graft, to create the tibial tunnel. A metal bone tunnel dilator (same size as before) is inserted in the tunnel and left in place to avoid interference between the tibial tunnel and the proximal anterior cancel-lous screw. The last screw is inserted; the dilatator is removed, and the shuttle suture is retrieved through the tibial tunnel. The graft is inserted into the joint using the shuttle suture. The right tension is obtained, and tibial fixation is performed at 20° of flexion with an interference screw (1 or 2 mm larger than the tibial tunnel). The arming sutures of the graft's tails are tied to the plate for additional fixation.

POSTOPERATIVE REGIMEN

Postoperative regimen depends mostly on the fixation method and presence of concomitant surgeries (ie, meniscal or cartilage procedures). Most of the investigators agree that, if a Puddu plate is used, patients should be kept partially or toe-touch weight-bearing in a hinged knee brace for 6 weeks (range 4–8 weeks).[1,4,15,20,44–46] However, some investigators allow for partial weight-bearing at 2 weeks after surgery and full weight-bearing at 4 weeks if a locking plate is used, with good results.[47]

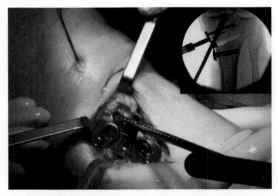

Fig. 5. The tibial aperture of the tunnel is performed anteriorly to the plate into the prox-imal tibial fragment. The guidewire is overdrilled with a cannulated reamer of the same size of the graft, to create the tibial tunnel. A metal bone tunnel dilator (same size as before) is then inserted in the tunnel and left in place to avoid interference between the tibial tunnel and the proximal anterior cancellous screw. On the right, a fluoroscopic image of the tunnel dilator inserted in the tibial tunnel.

Six weeks after surgery, a radiograph is performed, and, if osteotomy healing is confirmed, patients may be allowed progressive full weight-bearing, brace removal, and proceeding of rehabilitation program as in standard ACL-R.[15] At 12 weeks, another radiographic evaluation is normally performed, including long-leg view, to verify the alignment. Resumption of normal daily activities and even strenuous sports can be expected with significant differences in time between investigators.[45,48,49]

RESULTS

There are different studies in literature describing the outcomes of HTO combined with ACL-R/revision, mostly with a short follow-up period (mean of 5.25 years) and few recruited patients.[16,42,44,45,47–59] Furthermore, different HTO or ACL-R techniques are described in the literature, and the outcomes are difficult to compare. However, most of the studies concluded about improvement of the knee scores, such as International Knee Documentation Committee (IKDC) or Lysholm, as well as knee alignment and stability with good patient satisfaction after HTO combined to ACL-R/revision. These studies are summarized in **Table 2**. In most cases, concomitant HTO and ACL-R are performed in young and active patients, and the return to sport and preinjury level of activity is a concern. Trojani and colleagues,[49] in their study on 29 patients, concluded that 80% of the patients resumed sport activity, with 50% returning to competitive sport. Boss and colleagues[58] reported that 52% of the patients improved their sport activity level compared with the preoperative level, but it was still lower compared with the preinjury level in all patients. Akamatsu and colleagues[47] and Zaffagnini and colleagues[42] observed that only a small number of patients returned to the preinjury level of activity (25% and 18%, respectively). Noyes and colleagues[60] evaluated 41 patients with clinical improvement at 4.8 years of follow-up in terms of pain, swelling, giving way, and patient satisfaction. Ten out of 15 patients with advanced medial tibiofemoral arthrosis (subchondral bone exposure) had significant improvements in symptoms with no differences between isolated HTO and combined HTO and ACL-R. The investigators also evaluated the differences between isolated HTO and combined HTO and ACL-R, concluding about a decreased anterior-posterior displacement in favor of the combined procedure. Zaffagnini and colleagues[42] described the outcomes of CWHTO and combined ACL-R performed in 32 patients with an average follow-up of 6.5 years, with significant improvement in all the scores. At the radiological evaluation, 22% of patients showed medial arthritis progression. Arun and colleagues[54] evaluated 30 patients with a minimum of 2-years follow-up after combined OWHTO and ACL-R, correlating postoperative PTS to IKDC score. The investigators demonstrated that patients with a decrease in PTS greater than 5° had better functional scores. Mehl and colleagues[57] compared 52 patients who underwent isolated HTO (group 1) with 52 patients who underwent combined HTO and ACL-R (group 2). In both groups, there was a significant improvement in all the scores without differences within the groups in terms of clinical outcomes, progression of arthritis, and postoperative complications.

There are few systematic reviews in literature evaluating the outcome of combined HTO and ACL-R.[44,48,50] In all the studies, there was an improvement in knee scores (Lysholm and IKDC), with good correction of varus alignment (average 8.3°) and a complications rate ranging from 0% to 30%. Furthermore, there was no difference in terms of outcome between different surgical techniques (ie, bone tendon bone [BTB] vs gracilis-semitendinosus [G-ST] or OWHTO vs CWHTO) and between concomitant HTO and ACL-R or isolated HTO and delayed ACL-R.[44,50,57,60] All these studies concluded that combined HTO and ACL-R is a safe treatment of patients

Table 2
Summary of literature on high tibial osteotomy and anterior cruciate ligament reconstruction outcomes

Study, y	No. of Patients	Mean Age (y)	Study Groups	Type of HTO	Graft Type	Post Operative Protocol	Mean Follow-Up (y)	Postoperative Alignment	Scores	Outcome	Complications
Noyes et al,[60] 1993	16 out of 41	32	Group 1: HTO + ACLR Group 2: HTO + EA Group 3: HTO	CW	BTB auto	TTWB 4 wk, PWB 8 wk, FWB 12 wk	4.8	6 Varus knees 1 Valgus knee 9 Optimal alignment	Modified Noyes Score	Improved IKDC postoperatively	2 failures 2 nonunion 4 ACL-R revision
Boss et al,[58] 1995	27 out of 34	36	HTO + ACL-R	24 CW 3 OW	BTB auto and LAD	ROM exercise from the first day FWB after dimission	6.2	10° to 5° valgus	IKDC KT1000	IKDC was "Normal" or "nearly normal" for most of the patients. Average KT1000 difference 3 mm	6 stiffness 3 failures
Williams et al,[56] 2003	13 out of 25	33.5	Group 1: HTO + ACL-R Group 2: HTO + Delayed ACL-R	CW	2 BTB auto 2 H auto 9 BTB allo	N/A	3.2	8.2° valgus	Lysholm Tegner	Improvement of all the scores	N/A

Study	Patients	Age	Procedure	Osteotomy	Graft	Rehabilitation	Follow-up	Alignment	Outcome tools	Results	Complications
Bonin et al,[45] 2004	30 out of 40	30	HTO + ACL-R	CW and OW	BTB auto	NWB for 8 wk	12	3° valgus	IKDC KT1000	Improvement of postoperative IKDC. Few millimeter KT 1000 difference	1 patella baja 1 stiffness 4 wound problems 7 DVT
Akamatsu et al,[47] 2010	4	45	HTO + ACL-R	OW	H auto	PWB after 2 wk, FWB after 4 wk, return to sport after 6 mo	2.3	5° valgus	AKS Lysholm Tegner	Improvement of all the score. All cases KT 1000 difference <2 mm	N/A
Demange et al,[59] 2011	8	39.1	HTO + ACL-R	OW	H auto	NWB for 6 wk, PWB 2 wk, FWB after 8 wk Sports allowed after 8 mo	N/A	1.2° valgus	Subjective evaluation	Patients were satisfied with the operation and felt knees were more stable	1 superficial infection
Zaffagnini et al,[42] 2013	32	40.1	HTO + ACL-R	CW	H auto	Long-leg brace for the first 4 wk. Passive ROM 0°–90° allowed after 2 wk. TTWB for 4 wk	6.5	0.4°	KT1000 IKDC Tegner EQ-5D VAS	Average reduction tibial anterior displacement 2.2 mm (KT-1000) Improvement IKDC and Tegner score. Reduction VAS score, improvement EQ-5D	1 severe malalignment
Trojani et al,[49] 2014	29 out of 34	43	HTO + ACL-R	OW	H auto	NWB for 6 wk	6	2.5° valgus	IKDC VAS TELOS 150N	70% of patients were pain free at the end of follow-up. Normal TELOS translation in 24 out of 29 patients	N/A

(continued on next page)

Table 2
(continued)

Study, y	No. of Patients	Mean Age (y)	Study Groups	Type of HTO	Graft Type	Post Operative Protocol	Mean Follow-Up (y)	Postoperative Alignment	Scores	Outcome	Complications
Schuster et al,[53] 2016	23	47	HTO + ACL-R + CR	OW	12 BTB auto, 17 H auto	20 kg WB for 8 wk	6	2° valgus	KT1000, IKDC	Improvement IKDC. Side-to-side difference with KT100 changed from 7.8-1.3 mm	1 ACL-R revision 2 extension deficit
Arun et al,[54] 2016	26 out of 30	36.3	HTO + ACL-R	OW	H auto	N/A	6.23	N/A	IKDC, Lysholm	PTS decrease <5° related to lower improvement IKDC and Lysholm	N/A
Vaishya et al,[55] 2016	40 out of 46	37.3	HTO + ACL-R	OW	H auto	NWB for 2 wk. FWB at 6 wk	1.3	0.5° Varus	IKDC, KOOS	92.5% had no swelling and stiffness. Significant improvement IKDC and KOOS	1 loss of 20° flexion 2 delayed union
Mehl et al,[57] 2017	27	40.5	Group 1: HTO	25 CW, 28 OW	14 BTB auto, 3 BTB allo, 9 H auto	N/A	4	0.4° valgus	Lysholm, IKDC, KT2000, Kallagren Lawrence	92% of all patients were very satisfied. 81% reported an improvement of pain. Improvement in scores and KT 1000 in both groups	5 elective removals of the plate
	26	35.4	Group 2: HTO + ACLR				7.7	2.1° valgus			

Schuster et al,[53] 2016	50	48.9	HTO + ACL-R + CR	OW	H auto	PWB for 8 wk, without ROM limitation	5.6	2.2° valgus	IKDC	Improvement postoperative IKDC	4 deficit of ROM (3 resolved after arthrolysis). 1 superficial wound infection
Jin et al,[46] 2018	24	40.2	HTO + ACL-R	OW	H auto	Brace and NWB for 4 wk, then progressive FWB allowed	5.2	1.2 valgus	Lysholm Tegner	Lysholm score improved from 58.5-94 points. Tegner score increased from 4 to 5.3	2 medial meniscal damage 1 full-thickness cartilage on medial femoral condyle 3 hyperesthesia in proximal tibia 3 progression of medial OA

Abbreviations: AKS, American Knee Society Score; CR, chondral resurfacing; CW, closing wedge; EA, extra-articular reconstruction; FWB, full weight-bearing; H, hamstrings; KOOS, Knee Osteoarthritis Outcome Score; N/A, not applicable; NWB, no weight-bearing; OW, opening wedge; PWB, partial weight-bearing; TTWB, toe-touch weight-bearing.

suffering from medial OA and knee instability with the advantages of a single hospitalization and rehabilitation for 2 procedures and an acceptable complication rate.[50,54]

SUMMARY

Combined HTO and ACL-R is a demanding procedure for both patients and surgeons. However, with strict patient selection, good outcomes may be achieved in young patients. The primary indication to combined HTO and ACL-R is early medial-compartment OA (Ahlbäck I-III) associated with varus malalignment and ACL tear with symptomatic AP instability or failed ACL-R. The combined procedure may also be indicated in patients with failed ACL-R or revision due to increased PTS, or in the case of double or triple varus, or if another procedure, such as a meniscal transplant, may be necessary in an ACL-deficient varus knee.[21,25]

Preoperative evaluation should include a complete series of radiographs (AP, latero-lateral [LL], Merchant, and Rosenberg views), an MRI of the affected knee, as well as a complete clinical evaluation, including gait analysis.[1] There are different surgical techniques described to perform an HTO, including CWHTO and OWHTO, with no evidence of superiority of 1 technique over the others.[4] However, in most of the studies on combined HTO and ACL-R, an OWHTO is performed because it allows also for PTS modification.[19,20] Furthermore, for the ACL-R, a soft tissue graft is preferred in these cases.[15] If a combined procedure is performed, the osteotomy should be performed first in order not to damage the graft. The plate should be positioned more posteriorly compared with a standard HTO in order to avoid PTS increase and to leave more space for AM tunnel on the tibia. Postoperatively, complete weight-bearing is allowed between 4 and 8 postoperative weeks,[23] and ROM exercise may be started from the first day after surgery.[15,45,46,49,53,59] Most of the studies on combined HTO and ACL-R reported good outcomes at the midterm follow-up (average 5.2 years). However, the complication rate is not so low, ranging from 0% to 30%, including stiffness, loss of ROM, deep vein thrombosis, and need for plate removal.[16,55,57,58,60] In most cases, combined HTO and ACL-R is performed in young and active patients, and the return to sport may be a concern. Most of the investigators described good return to sport rate, with few patients returning to competitive sports or to the preinjury level of activity.[42,49] In conclusion, combined HTO and ACL-R/revision may be a viable option in young patients affected by anterior instability and medial OA, with good midterm outcomes if a correct indication, preoperative planning, and surgical technique are applied.

REFERENCES

1. Rossi R, Bonasia DE, Amendola A. The role of high tibial osteotomy in the varus knee. J Am Acad Orthop Surg 2011;19:590–9.
2. O'Neill DF, James SL. Valgus osteotomy with anterior cruciate ligament laxity. Clin Orthop Relat Res 1992;(278):153–9.
3. Dejour H, Neyret P, Boileau P, et al. Anterior cruciate reconstruction combined with valgus tibial osteotomy. Clin Orthop Relat Res 1994;(299):220–8.
4. Amendola A, Bonasia DE. Results of high tibial osteotomy: review of the literature. Int Orthop 2010;34:155–60.
5. Brouwer RW, Bierma-Zeinstra SMA, van Raaij TM, et al. Osteotomy for medial compartment arthritis of the knee using a closing wedge or an opening wedge controlled by a Puddu plate. A one-year randomised, controlled study. J Bone Joint Surg Br 2006;88:1454–9.

6. Noyes FR, Barber-Westin SD, Hewett TE. High tibial osteotomy and ligament reconstruction for varus angulated anterior cruciate ligament-deficient knees. Am J Sports Med 2000;28:282–96.

7. Schipplein OD, Andriacchi TP. Interaction between active and passive knee stabilizers during level walking. J Orthop Res 1991;9:113–9.

8. Hughston JC, Jacobson KE. Chronic posterolateral rotatory instability of the knee. J Bone Joint Surg Am 1985;67:351–9.

9. Dugdale TW, Noyes FR, Styer D. Preoperative planning for high tibial osteotomy. The effect of lateral tibiofemoral separation and tibiofemoral length. Clin Orthop 1992;(274):248–64.

10. Noyes FR, Dunworth LA, Andriacchi TP, et al. Knee hyperextension gait abnormalities in unstable knees. Recognition and preoperative gait retraining. Am J Sports Med 1996;24:35–45.

11. Noyes FR, Schipplein OD, Andriacchi TP, et al. The anterior cruciate ligament-deficient knee with varus alignment. An analysis of gait adaptations and dynamic joint loadings. Am J Sports Med 1992;20:707–16.

12. Dejour H, Bonnin M. Tibial translation after anterior cruciate ligament rupture. Two radiological tests compared. J Bone Joint Surg Br 1994;76:745–9.

13. Herman BV, Giffin JR. High tibial osteotomy in the ACL-deficient knee with medial compartment osteoarthritis. J Orthop Traumatol 2016;17:277–85.

14. Genin P, Weill G, Julliard R. The tibial slope. Proposal for a measurement method. J Radiol 1993;74:27–33 [in French].

15. Bonasia DE, Dettoni F, Palazzolo A, et al. Opening wedge high tibial osteotomy and anterior cruciate ligament reconstruction or revision. Arthrosc Tech 2017;6: e1735–41.

16. Schuster P, Geßlein M, Schlumberger M, et al. The influence of tibial slope on the graft in combined high tibial osteotomy and anterior cruciate ligament reconstruction. Knee 2018;25:682–91.

17. Brouwer RW, Bierma-Zeinstra SMA, van Koeveringe AJ, et al. Patellar height and the inclination of the tibial plateau after high tibial osteotomy: the open *versus* the closed-wedge technique. J Bone Joint Surg Br 2005;87-B:1227–32.

18. Hohmann E, Bryant A, Reaburn P, et al. Is there a correlation between posterior tibial slope and non-contact anterior cruciate ligament injuries? Knee Surg Sports Traumatol Arthrosc 2011;19:109–14.

19. Noyes FR, Goebel SX, West J. Opening wedge tibial osteotomy: the 3-triangle method to correct axial alignment and tibial slope. Am J Sports Med 2005;33: 378–87.

20. Savarese E, Bisicchia S, Romeo R, et al. Role of high tibial osteotomy in chronic injuries of posterior cruciate ligament and posterolateral corner. J Orthop Traumatol 2011;12:1–17.

21. Won HH, Chang CB, Je MS, et al. Coronal limb alignment and indications for high tibial osteotomy in patients undergoing revision ACL reconstruction. Clin Orthop 2013;471:3504–11.

22. Markolf KL, Bargar WL, Shoemaker SC, et al. The role of joint load in knee stability. J Bone Joint Surg Am 1981;63:570–85.

23. Loia MC, Vanni S, Rosso F, et al. High tibial osteotomy in varus knees: indications and limits. Joints 2016;4:98–110.

24. Kim S-J, Moon H-K, Chun Y-M, et al. Is correctional osteotomy crucial in primary varus knees undergoing anterior cruciate ligament reconstruction? Clin Orthop 2011;469:1421–6.

25. Bonasia DE, Amendola A. Combined medial meniscal transplantation and high tibial osteotomy. Knee Surg Sports Traumatol Arthrosc 2010;18:870–3.
26. Badhe NP, Forster IW. High tibial osteotomy in knee instability: the rationale of treatment and early results. Knee Surg Sports Traumatol Arthrosc 2002;10:38–43.
27. Ranawat AS, Nwachukwu BU, Pearle AD, et al. Comparison of lateral closing-wedge versus medial opening-wedge high tibial osteotomy on knee joint alignment and kinematics in the ACL-deficient knee. Am J Sports Med 2016;44:3103–10.
28. Trieb K, Grohs J, Hanslik-Schnabel B, et al. Age predicts outcome of high-tibial osteotomy. Knee Surg Sports Traumatol Arthrosc 2006;14:149–52.
29. Rudan JF, Simurda MA. High tibial osteotomy. A prospective clinical and roentgenographic review. Clin Orthop 1990;(255):251–6.
30. Marriott K, Birmingham TB, Kean CO, et al. Five-year changes in gait biomechanics after concomitant high tibial osteotomy and ACL reconstruction in patients with medial knee osteoarthritis. Am J Sports Med 2015;43:2277–85.
31. Chang A, Hayes K, Dunlop D, et al. Thrust during ambulation and the progression of knee osteoarthritis. Arthritis Rheum 2004;50:3897–903.
32. Sharma L, Chang AH, Jackson RD, et al. Varus thrust and incident and progressive knee osteoarthritis. Arthritis Rheumatol 2017;69:2136–43.
33. Lee DC, Byun SJ. High tibial osteotomy. Knee Surg Relat Res 2012;24:61–9.
34. Naudie DDR, Amendola A, Fowler PJ. Opening wedge high tibial osteotomy for symptomatic hyperextension-varus thrust. Am J Sports Med 2004;32:60–70.
35. Miller MD, Cole BJ, Cosgarea A. Operative techniques: sports knee surgery. In: Sekiya JK, editor. Operative techniques: sports knee surgery. 1 Har/DVD edition. Philadelphia: Saunders; 2008. p. 544. Hardcover.
36. Li Y, Hong L, Feng H, et al. Posterior tibial slope influences static anterior tibial translation in anterior cruciate ligament reconstruction: a minimum 2-year follow-up study. Am J Sports Med 2014;42:927–33.
37. Rodner CM, Adams DJ, Diaz-Doran V, et al. Medial opening wedge tibial osteotomy and the sagittal plane: the effect of increasing tibial slope on tibiofemoral contact pressure. Am J Sports Med 2006;34:1431–41.
38. Marti CB, Gautier E, Wachtl SW, et al. Accuracy of frontal and sagittal plane correction in open-wedge high tibial osteotomy. Arthroscopy 2004;20:366–72.
39. Phillips CL, Silver D a T, Schranz PJ, et al. The measurement of patellar height: a review of the methods of imaging. J Bone Joint Surg Br 2010;92:1045–53.
40. Imhoff AB, Agneskirchner J. Simultaneous ACL replacement and high tibial osteotomy: indication, technique, results. Tech Knee Surg 2002;1:146–54.
41. Amendola A. Unicompartmental osteoarthritis in the active patient: the role of high tibial osteotomy. Arthroscopy 2003;19(Suppl 1):109–16.
42. Zaffagnini S, Bonanzinga T, Grassi A, et al. Combined ACL reconstruction and closing-wedge HTO for varus angulated ACL-deficient knees. Knee Surg Sports Traumatol Arthrosc 2013;21:934–41.
43. Gomoll AH, Filardo G, Almqvist FK, et al. Surgical treatment for early osteoarthritis. Part II: allografts and concurrent procedures. Knee Surg Sports Traumatol Arthrosc 2012;20:468–86.
44. Crawford MD, Diehl LH, Amendola A. Surgical management and treatment of the anterior cruciate ligament-deficient knee with malalignment. Clin Sports Med 2017;36:119–33.
45. Bonin N, Ait Si Selmi T, Donell ST, et al. Anterior cruciate reconstruction combined with valgus upper tibial osteotomy: 12 years follow-up. Knee 2004;11:431–7.

46. Jin C, Song E-K, Jin Q-H, et al. Outcomes of simultaneous high tibial osteotomy and anterior cruciate ligament reconstruction in anterior cruciate ligament deficient knee with osteoarthritis. BMC Musculoskelet Disord 2018;19:228.

47. Akamatsu Y, Mitsugi N, Taki N, et al. Simultaneous anterior cruciate ligament reconstruction and opening wedge high tibial osteotomy: report of four cases. Knee 2010;17:114–8.

48. Li Y, Zhang H, Zhang J, et al. Clinical outcome of simultaneous high tibial osteotomy and anterior cruciate ligament reconstruction for medial compartment osteoarthritis in young patients with anterior cruciate ligament-deficient knees: a systematic review. Arthroscopy 2015;31:507–19.

49. Trojani C, Elhor H, Carles M, et al. Anterior cruciate ligament reconstruction combined with valgus high tibial osteotomy allows return to sports. Orthop Traumatol Surg Res 2014;100:213–6.

50. Malahias M-A, Shahpari O, Kaseta M-K. The clinical outcome of one-stage high tibial osteotomy and anterior cruciate ligament reconstruction. A current concept systematic and comprehensive review. Arch Bone Jt Surg 2018;6:161–8.

51. Cantin O, Magnussen RA, Corbi F, et al. The role of high tibial osteotomy in the treatment of knee laxity: a comprehensive review. Knee Surg Sports Traumatol Arthrosc 2015;23:3026–37.

52. Mancuso F, Hamilton TW, Kumar V, et al. Clinical outcome after UKA and HTO in ACL deficiency: a systematic review. Knee Surg Sports Traumatol Arthrosc 2016; 24:112–22.

53. Schuster P, Schulz M, Richter J. Combined biplanar high tibial osteotomy, anterior cruciate ligament reconstruction, and abrasion/microfracture in severe medial osteoarthritis of unstable varus knees. Arthroscopy 2016;32:283–92.

54. Arun GR, Kumaraswamy V, Rajan D, et al. Long-term follow up of single-stage anterior cruciate ligament reconstruction and high tibial osteotomy and its relation with posterior tibial slope. Arch Orthop Trauma Surg 2016;136:505–11.

55. Vaishya R, Vijay V, Jha GK, et al. Prospective study of the anterior cruciate ligament reconstruction associated with high tibial opening wedge osteotomy in knee arthritis associated with instability. J Clin Orthop Trauma 2016;7:265–71.

56. Williams RJ, Kelly BT, Wickiewicz TL, et al. The short-term outcome of surgical treatment for painful varus arthritis in association with chronic ACL deficiency. J Knee Surg 2003;16:9–16.

57. Mehl J, Paul J, Feucht MJ, et al. ACL deficiency and varus osteoarthritis: high tibial osteotomy alone or combined with ACL reconstruction? Arch Orthop Trauma Surg 2017;137:233–40.

58. Boss A, Stutz G, Oursin C, et al. Anterior cruciate ligament reconstruction combined with valgus tibial osteotomy (combined procedure). Knee Surg Sports Traumatol Arthrosc 1995;3:187–91.

59. Demange MK, Camanho GL, Pécora JR, et al. Simultaneous anterior cruciate ligament reconstruction and computer-assisted open-wedge high tibial osteotomy: a report of eight cases. Knee 2011;18:387–91.

60. Noyes FR, Barber SD, Simon R. High tibial osteotomy and ligament reconstruction in varus angulated, anterior cruciate ligament-deficient knees: a two- to seven-year follow-up study. Am J Sports Med 1993;21:2–12.

The Role of Osteotomy in Chronic Valgus Instability and Hyperextension Valgus Thrust (Medial Closing Wedge Distal Femoral Varus Osteotomy and Lateral Opening Wedge High Tibial Osteotomy)

Philip P. Roessler, MD, Alan Getgood, MPhil, MD, FRCS(Tr&Orth)*

KEYWORDS

- Valgus instability • Valgus thrust • Valgus malalignment • Osteotomy • HTO • DFVO

KEY POINTS

- Chronic valgus instability and concomitant valgus malalignment together pose a situation that cannot be controlled by ligament surgery alone.
- Hyperextension valgus thrust is a relatively rare phenomenon that can occur in cases of combined instability and malalignment.
- Osteotomies around the knee (medial closing wedge distal femoral varus osteotomy and lateral opening wedge high tibial osteotomy) are an option to treat both conditions with or without concomitant ligament surgery at the medial side to normalize the mechanical leg axis and relieve instability.
- In cases of multiligament instability with concomitant valgus malalignment, additional varus osteotomies are an option to reduce the risks of early graft failure (eg, anterior cruciate ligament/posterior cruciate ligament), by restoring near physiologic kinematics.

INTRODUCTION

The medial side of the knee consists of various distinct anatomic structures. The medial collateral ligament (MCL) is considered as one of the main static stabilizers of the knee joint and is also among the most commonly injured structures. It is divided into a superficial (sMCL) and deep (dMCL) portion. Besides the

Fowler Kennedy Sports Medicine Clinic, Western University, 1151 Richmond Street, London, Ontario N6A 3K7, Canada
* Corresponding author.
E-mail address: alan.getgood@uwo.ca

MCL, there are other static structures including the posterior oblique ligament (POL) that resides within the posteromedial capsule, and dynamic structures, such as the hamstring tendons, all of which add to the stability of the medial aspect of the knee.[1] Although treatment options for most medial-sided injuries evolve toward nonoperative management, early and sufficient treatment is still advised. If not treated properly, acute injuries of the medial side may lead to chronic valgus instability.[2]

Chronic valgus instability results from an unhealed MCL tear or avulsion with subsequent laxity on the medial side.[3,4] Chronicity, in this context, has been defined as 12 weeks past acute injury.[5] Various other factors may cause or influence instability. Among them is stability of the anterior cruciate ligament/posterior cruciate ligament (ACL/PCL) or individual bony morphology.[2] Clinically, most patients suffer from combined medial and lateral-sided pain, as well as subjective instability and giving-way preventing them from physical activity or sports. Although the sMCL is best tested in 30° of flexion, there may also be instability in extension or hyperextension, indicating involvement of the ACL/PCL or the POL.[4] In these cases, valgus thrust is seen as a common clinical sign of chronic instability of the medial side.

In comparison to varus thrust, the valgus thrust phenomenon is relatively rare with a prevalence of approximately 7% in individuals without and 9% with radiographic signs of osteoarthritis (OA).[6] Its mechanism is defined as a dynamic increase of (preexisting) valgus during the stance phase, followed by a decrease during the lift-off and swing phases of gait.[6] Because the lateral tibial plateau literally smashes against the lateral femoral condyle during valgus thrust, lateral compartment load transmission and contact pressures may increase drastically. This mechanism has been identified as a potential cause of lateral compartment OA progression. Valgus thrust can be caused by either capsuloligamentous (eg, valgus instability) or neuromuscular (eg, quadriceps weakness) insufficiency. Depending on its etiology, there are primary and secondary forms. Obesity may be an additional factor, due to increased axial load on the knee joint and wide stance gait secondary to the increased soft tissue envelope. Preexisting innate or secondary valgus malalignment in the frontal plane has been identified as the most important risk factor for valgus thrust.[6]

Treatment options for chronic valgus instability are based on anatomic considerations. Besides ligamentous reconstruction of the MCL, tightening of the medial structures including the POL and the posterior capsule has been proposed.[7] In combination injuries of MCL and ACL, multiligament reconstruction procedures also may be necessary.[8] Cases of chronic valgus instability with an additional valgus malalignment in the frontal plane on the other hand require deformity correction by osteotomies rather than sole soft tissue surgery alone.

INDICATIONS

Chronic valgus instability with an additional valgus malalignment may cause symptomatic lateral compartment overload, eventually leading to selective unicompartmental OA. In this context, valgus malalignment is defined as a weight-bearing line crossing the lateral tibial spine toward the lateral compartment or greater than 10° of valgus malalignment of the mechanical axis in the frontal plane.[9] Ligamentous reconstruction of the medial aspect of the knee alone normally does not resolve symptoms, especially those caused by progressive OA, as it only addresses one aspect of this combined pathology. Those cases pose a primary indication for osteotomies around the knee. As for most forms of bony valgus malalignment, femoral correction via a biplanar medial closing wedge distal femoral varus osteotomy (MCWDFVO) is the authors' preferred technique here, although tibial correction via a lateral opening wedge high tibial osteotomy (LOWHTO) can be done for smaller degrees of correction. However, due to a certain risk of later joint line obliquity, varus high tibial osteotomy (HTO) appears to be less preferential.[10] Although it can be done simultaneously, additional soft tissue surgery (if still needed) is done after consolidation of these procedures and return to activity.[9]

Relative contraindications for either HTO or distal femoral varus osteotomy (DFVO) in cases of combined chronic valgus instability and valgus malalignment include tricompartmental OA, extreme valgus deformity with tibial subluxation, multidirectional instabilities, flexion contracture >15°, high body mass index (>30 kg/m^2), rheumatoid arthritis, and severe bone loss at the lateral compartment.[11]

PREOPERATIVE PLANNING

- Clinical evaluation
  - Physical examination to evaluate pain focus, extent of joint laxity, valgus thrust phenomenon (if present) during gait, limb alignment in frontal and sagittal planes (eg, genu valgum).
  - Tests for knee laxity (Lachman, anterior and posterior drawer, pivot shift and reverse pivot shift, rotational combined tests) to rule out pathology other than valgus laxity
- Radiographs
  - Bilateral weight-bearing long-leg standing (hip-to-ankle) a.p (**Fig. 1**).
  - Bilateral weight-bearing Rosenberg's view posteroanterior (**Fig. 2**A).
  - Bilateral standard anteroposterior in full extension (**Fig. 2**B), horizontal beam lateral (**Fig. 2**C) and patella sunrise views
  - Optional: Bilateral stress radiographs a.p. to be able to subtract the degree of deformity caused by ligamentous valgus laxity during planning (**Fig. 3**)
- Advanced imaging
  - MRI of the involved knee to confirm medial-sided injury or scarring and rule out concomitant pathologies like ACL/PCL, meniscal, or chondral injuries
  - Optional: Rotational profile computed tomography to rule out torsional deformities
- Further considerations
  - Isolated chronic valgus instability without concomitant (mostly ACL) injury is regarded very rare. For this reason, sole treatment with osteotomy requires a strict indication and ruling out all important cofactors of instability as mentioned previously.
  - Preexisting valgus malalignment may complicate or even hinder nonoperative treatment of medial side injuries. For this reason, early operative treatment with alignment correction is advisable.
- Planning of LOWHTO
  - Typically done according to Dugdale and colleagues (**Fig. 4**).[12]
  - Indication: Valgus deformity secondary to intra-articular deformity that is meniscus/articular cartilage loss
  - Anatomic axis of femur should be normal
  - Correction will be achieved through full flexion arc, unlike MCWDFVO, which will work primarily in extension
  - Resultant correction will not create a joint line obliquity greater than 10°

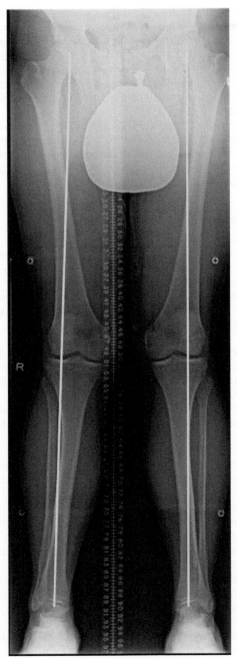

Fig. 1. Bilateral weight-bearing long-leg standing (hip-to-ankle) a.p. to verify valgus malalignment in the coronal plane. The patient can be assessed for side-to-side differences and weight-bearing conditions ensure that even functional malalignment of the lower extremities is detected.

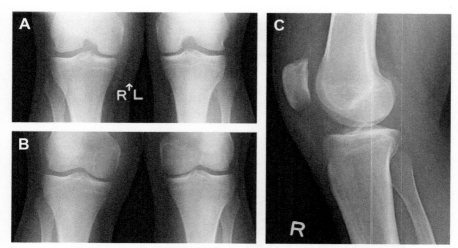

Fig. 2. (*A*) Bilateral weight-bearing Rosenberg's view p.a. (*B*) Bilateral standard a.p. in full extension. (*C*) Horizontal beam lateral. These standard radiographs help to identify joint line obliquity, posterior tibial slope and side-to-side differences in bony morphology. The Rosenberg's view will help to estimate the degree of joint space narrowing or OA in the main weight-bearing zone of the femoral condyles.

- Planning of MCWDFVO
  - Typically done according to Dugdale and colleagues (see **Fig. 4**).[12]
  - Desired weight-bearing line between center of knee to tip of medial tibial spine
  - No overcorrection to varus to avoid overload OA

PREPARATION AND POSITIONING

- Supine position on radiolucent/carbon table
- Additional lateral post lateral to the proximal thigh as a bolster for intraoperative stress testing as well as footrest to enable a position of 30° flexion
- Tourniquet around proximal thigh (300 mm Hg)
- C-arm/fluoroscopy with sterile draping for intraoperative controls
- Single-shot antibiotics following individual protocol for bone surgery

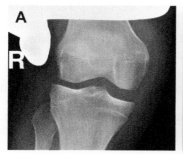
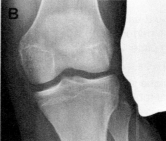

Fig. 3. Bilateral stress radiographs a.p. will help to estimate side-to-side differences in valgus instability (in this case 5 mm right [*A*] to left [*B*]) and subtract its addition to the degree of deformity during later planning of the osteotomy.

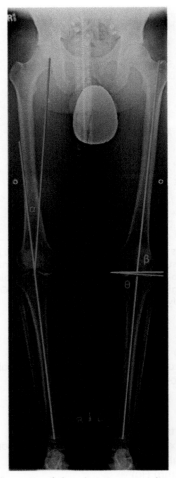

α – Mechanical Tibiofemoral
Angle (mTFA)
(normal = 1.3° +/- 2°)

B – Anatomic Lateral Distal
Femoral Angle (aLDFA)
(normal = 81° +/- 2°)

Θ – Anatomic Medial Proximal
Tibial Angle (aMPTA)
(normal = 87° +/- 2°)

Δ – Proximal Posterior Tibial
Articular Angle (PPTA)
(normal = 81° +/- 3°)

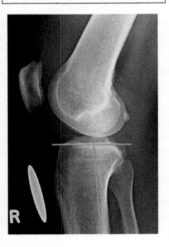

Fig. 4. Schematic of the planning according to Dugdale.

SURGICAL TECHNIQUE (STEP-BY-STEP DESCRIPTION OF THE SURGICAL PROCEDURE; PLEASE USE SURGICAL IMAGES)

The following 2 easy stepwise procedures are the authors' preferred techniques and can easily be performed using standard AO instruments and special anatomic osteotomy locking plates.

- LOWHTO
  1. Oblique skin incision between the anterior portion of the fibular head and the tibial tubercle (**Fig. 5**).
  2. Tibialis anterior is elevated off the tibia back to the anterior joint capsule of the proximal tibiofibular joint, which is then incised and opened to mobilize it to avoid any restrictions for the following tibial osteotomy (**Fig. 6**).
  3. The patellar tendon is then secured by a blunt Hohmann retractor, as is the posterior aspect of the tibia to protect neurovascular structures, before insertion of the guide pin for the osteotomy (**Fig. 7**).

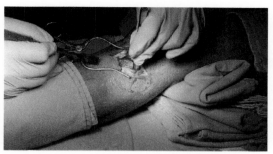

Fig. 5. Oblique skin incision.

4. Pin position is checked with fluoroscopy. The tip should be aiming at the desired medial hinge and the guide pin should recreate the direction of the osteotomy cut (**Fig. 8**).
5. Biplanar tibial osteotomy is performed with an oscillating saw first creating an up-cut tibial tubercle osteotomy (TTO) and then starting the tibial osteotomy cut as shown and cautiously completing it with an osteotome under fluoroscopic guidance to avoid inadvertent neurovascular injuries (**Fig. 9**).
6. The osteotomy is then opened with a distracting osteotome and temporarily held in place with a lamina spreader (**Fig. 10**).
7. After inserting the submuscular HTO locking plate and fixing it with proper screws under fluoroscopic guidance, the lamina spreader can be removed again (**Fig. 11**).
8. Final fluoroscopic assessment will help to check for the desired degree of correction in the coronal plane as well as correct screw placement (**Fig. 12**).
- MCWDFVO
  1. Medial skin incision (**Fig. 13**).
  2. Subvastus approach and elevating muscle off the septum and securing it with a blunt Hohmann retractor anteriorly and posteriorly (**Fig. 14**).
  3. Insertion of the guide pins at the proximal and distal osteotomy and checking their trajectory with fluoroscopy. Care has to be taken not to produce a cortical mismatch between both, proximal and distal, osteotomies, especially in terms of length (**Fig. 15**).
  4. Biplanar femoral osteotomy is performed with an oscillating saw as shown starting with the distal osteotomy, then moving forward to the proximal

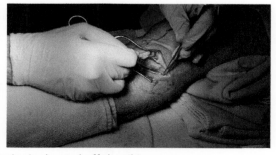

Fig. 6. Tibialis anterior is elevated off the tibia.

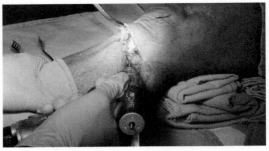

Fig. 7. Securing of patellar tendon and posterior tibia before guide pin insertion.

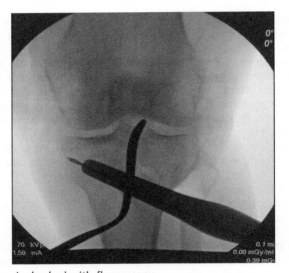

Fig. 8. Pin position is checked with fluoroscopy.

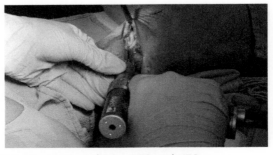

Fig. 9. Biplanar tibial osteotomy combining TTO and HTO.

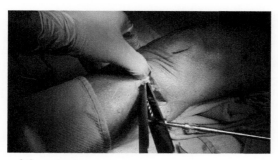

Fig. 10. Distraction of the osteotomy.

osteotomy, completing both with an osteotome to avoid neurovascular injuries at the medial side. An additional coronal plane osteotomy (dotted line) has to be completed anteriorly to allow for gentle removal of the wedge. Care has to be taken not to harm the trochlea in this procedure (**Fig. 16**).

5. The osteotomy is closed gently and gradually to avoid hinge fractures. A controlled osteoclasis of the lateral hinge may be performed to weaken the cortical bridge without fracturing, using a 2.4-mm pin. The submuscular DFVO locking plate is then inserted anteromedially to ensure good coverage by the muscular tissue and reduce later mechanical irritation. To secure the plate, screws are inserted and fixed starting with the distal ones. Final fluoroscopic assessment will help to check for the desired degree of correction in the coronal plane as well as correct screw placement (**Fig. 17**).

COMPLICATIONS

Besides the general complication profile of bone surgery on the lower extremities, several complications specific to HTO and DFVO have been reported in the literature.

- Lateral hinge fractures or intra-articular tibial plateau fractures in HTO
- Medial hinge factures or distal femoral fractures in DFVO
- Neurovascular injury
- Hardware failure with subsequent loss of correction
- Mechanical irritation due to hardware
- Surgical site infection
- Nonunion or delayed union

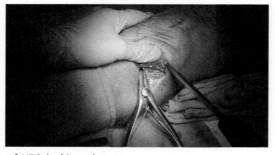

Fig. 11. Placement of HTO locking plate.

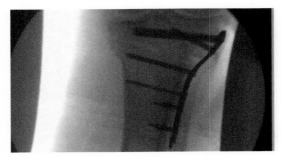

Fig. 12. Final fluoroscopic assessment.

POSTOPERATIVE REGIMEN

- Toe touch weight-bearing for the initial 2 weeks postoperatively.
- If performed, concomitant ligament reconstruction will then dictate rehabilitation. If the MCL is reconstructed, partial weight bearing is mandated from 2 to 6 weeks postoperative in the range-of-motion brace.
- If osteotomy performed alone, then weight-bearing as tolerated is allowed starting from week 3 postoperatively.
- Hinged knee brace for 6 weeks postoperatively.
- Thrombosis prophylaxis with low molecular-weight heparin for 6 weeks postoperatively.
- Range-of-motion exercised immediately postoperatively in brace.
- Return to activity 12 weeks postoperatively (low impact) and 24 weeks postoperatively (high impact).

RESULTS

Although a significant amount of data exists in the present literature pertaining to osteotomies for chronic varus instability or hyperextension varus thrust,[13–15] there is minimal data available with regard to osteotomies for valgus instability or hyperextension valgus thrust.

Cameron and Saha[16] report good alignment correction in 34 of 35 patients with the MCL still being lax following osteotomy but without functional restrictions or a need for secondary procedures. Accordingly, Phisitkul and colleagues[9] report that only occasionally secondary ligamentous procedures are required in very active patients or athletes.

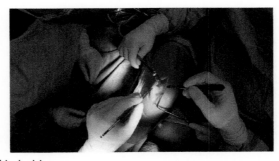

Fig. 13. Medial skin incision.

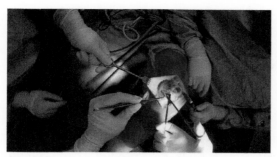

Fig. 14. Subvastus approach.

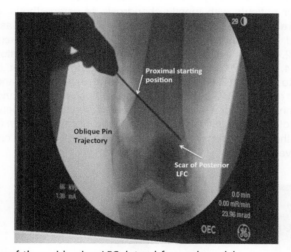

Fig. 15. Insertion of the guide pins. LFC, lateral femoral condyle.

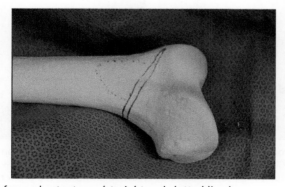

Fig. 16. Biplanar femoral osteotomy (*straight* and *dotted lines*).

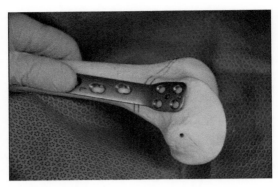

Fig. 17. Placement of DFVO locking plate.

Collins and colleagues[17] report midterm results of LOWHTO in 24 cases of valgus malalignment for patients with mostly chondrosis or osteoarthritis. Significant improvements were identified in the lower extremity functional scale as well as in the knee injury and osteoarthritis outcome score. The mechanical axis significantly changed from 2.4 ± 2.4° valgus to 0 ± 2.6° varus and the anatomic axis from 6.9 ± 2.8° to 4.7 ± 2.5° valgus, with weight-bearing line offset changing from 60.2 ± 11.4% to 49.5 ± 12.4%. In a systematic review, Saithna and colleagues[18] report long-term results of MCWDFVO in 130 pooled patients with various indications of valgus malalignment. After a follow-up of 10 years, survival rates between 64% and 82% could be noted with significant (and sustained) improvements in functional knee scores such as the hospital for special surgery score. In most of the cases, hardware had to be removed again.

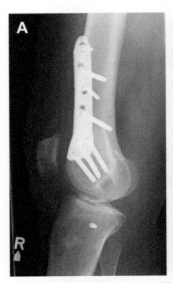
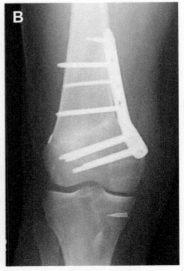

Fig. 18. (A) Horizontal beam lateral and (B) standard a.p. in full extension 10 months after staged PCL + MCL and ACL + lateral meniscus posterior root repair + MCWDFVO. No hardware-associated complication could be recorded and there is a proper union at the osteotomy site.

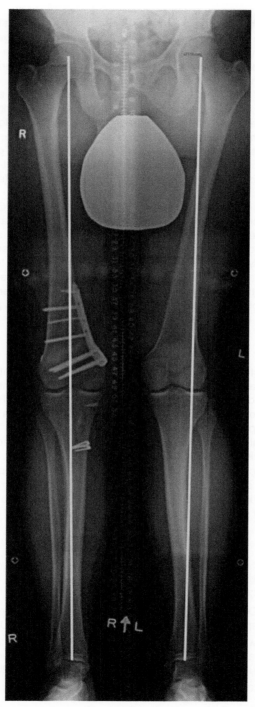

Fig. 19. Neutral alignment of the involved right side (as compared with the contralateral left side) 10 months after staged PCL + MCL and ACL + lateral meniscus posterior root repair + MCWDFVO.

We present a case of a 22-year-old man 2 months following right knee injury during sporting activity. He was riding a pedal bike, lost control over a large ramp, and dropped 3 to 5 m deep twisting his knee. The patient was treated with a locking extension brace in the emergency department. Besides his injuries, there were no other health-related issues and no ongoing medication or medical treatment.

After 7 weeks, he presented himself at our outpatient clinic with a subjective instability of his involved (right) knee joint ("inside of knee opens up during walking"). Clinically he showed a tenderness at the medial joint line as well as a valgus alignment with a positive valgus thrust during gait. His Beighton Score was greater than 5, indicating general ligamentous laxity. On specific examination he exhibited a grade 3 PCL laxity and a grade 3 MCL laxity as well as a grade 2 Lachman and pivot-shift tests. These findings could be confirmed in plain radiographic assessment (see **Figs. 1–3**) as well as MRI.

The patient was treated in a staged approach, first repairing his PCL and MCL with a tibialis anterior allograft, additionally reinforcing the POL with a fiber tape. After 6 weeks of protected weight-bearing, his ACL was repaired with a tibialis posterior allograft in a second stage, additionally repairing the lateral meniscus posterior root and performing an MCWDFVO to correct his valgus malalignment to protect the ligament grafts. After an additional 6 weeks of protected weight-bearing, the patient returned to occupational duties and resumed sporting activity after 10 months. Plain radiographic controls showed a good position of the hardware, a proper union, and a neutral alignment on the involved right side (**Figs. 18** and **19**).

SUMMARY

Chronic valgus instability with concomitant valgus malalignment remains a challenging diagnosis, as it cannot be successfully treated with ligament surgery alone. Osteotomies around the knee, especially MCWDFVO and LOWHTO, provide an option to deal with both issues by normalizing the mechanical axis of the femur and thus reducing symptoms of chronic valgus instability like valgus thrust. In most of the cases of sole valgus instability, additional ligament surgery is required only if there is a residual subjective or objective instability afterward. In complex cases of multiligament injuries with concomitant valgus malalignment, osteotomies are an option to reduce the risks of early graft failure (eg, ACL/PCL) by reducing in situ forces on the ligamentous structures. Altogether, osteotomies around the knee are an additional means of treatment in complex knee surgery dealing with cases of chronic instability.

REFERENCES

1. LaPrade MD, Kennedy MI, Wijdicks CA, et al. Anatomy and biomechanics of the medial side of the knee and their surgical implications. Sports Med Arthrosc Rev 2015;23(2):63–70.
2. Chen L, Kim PD, Ahmad CS, et al. Medial collateral ligament injuries of the knee: current treatment concepts. Curr Rev Musculoskelet Med 2008;1(2):108–13.
3. Robins AJ, Newman AP, Burks RT. Postoperative return of motion in anterior cruciate ligament and medial collateral ligament injuries. The effect of medial collateral ligament rupture location. Am J Sports Med 1993;21(1):20–5.
4. Indelicato P. Isolated medial collateral ligament injuries in the knee. J Am Acad Orthop Surg 1995;3(1):9–14.
5. Slocum DB, Larson RL, James SL. Late reconstruction procedures used to stabilize the knee. Orthop Clin North Am 1973;4(3):679–89.

6. Chang A, Hochberg M, Song J, et al. Frequency of varus and valgus thrust and factors associated with thrust presence in persons with or at higher risk of developing knee osteoarthritis. Arthritis Rheum 2010;62(5):1403–11.
7. Paley D, Bhatnagar J, Herzenberg JE, et al. New procedures for tightening knee collateral ligaments in conjunction with knee realignment osteotomy. Orthop Clin North Am 1994;25(3):533–55. Available at: http://eutils.ncbi.nlm.nih.gov/entrez/eutils/elink.fcgi?dbfrom=pubmed&id=8028894&retmode=ref&cmd=prlinks.
8. Bonasia DE, Bruzzone M, Dettoni F, et al. Treatment of medial and posteromedial knee instability: indications, techniques, and review of the results. Iowa Orthop J 2012;32:173–83.
9. Phisitkul P, Wolf BR, Amendola A. Role of high tibial and distal femoral osteotomies in the treatment of lateral-posterolateral and medial instabilities of the knee. Sports Med Arthrosc Rev 2006;14(2):96–104.
10. Jiang KN, West RV. Management of chronic combined ACL medial posteromedial instability of the knee. Sports Med Arthrosc Rev 2015;23(2):85–90.
11. Cole BJ, Sekiya JK. Surgical techniques of the shoulder, elbow and knee in sports medicine E-book. Philadelphia: Elsevier Health Sciences; 2013.
12. Dugdale TW, Noyes FR, Styer D. Preoperative planning for high tibial osteotomy. The effect of lateral tibiofemoral separation and tibiofemoral length. Clin Orthop Relat Res 1992;274:248–64. Available at: http://eutils.ncbi.nlm.nih.gov/entrez/eutils/elink.fcgi?dbfrom=pubmed&id=1729010&retmode=ref&cmd=prlinks.
13. Naudie DDR, Amendola A, Fowler PJ. Opening wedge high tibial osteotomy for symptomatic hyperextension-varus thrust. Am J Sports Med 2004;32(1):60–70.
14. Gardiner A, Gutiérrez Sevilla GR, Steiner ME, et al. Osteotomies about the knee for tibiofemoral malalignment in the athletic patient. Am J Sports Med 2010;38(5):1038–47.
15. Cantin O, Magnussen RA, Corbi F, et al. The role of high tibial osteotomy in the treatment of knee laxity: a comprehensive review. Knee Surg Sports Traumatol Arthrosc 2015;23(10):3026–37.
16. Cameron JC, Saha S. Management of medial collateral ligament laxity. Orthop Clin North Am 1994;25(3):527–32.
17. Collins B, Getgood AM, Alomar AZ, et al. A case series of lateral opening wedge high tibial osteotomy for valgus malalignment. Knee Surg Sports Traumatol Arthrosc 2013;21(1):152–60.
18. Saithna A, Kundra R, Modi CS, et al. Distal femoral varus osteotomy for lateral compartment osteoarthritis in the valgus knee. A systematic review of the literature. Open Orthop J 2012;6(1):313–9.

The Use of Navigation in Osteotomies Around the Knee

Thomas Neri, MD, PhD*, Darli Myat, PhD, David Parker, BMedSci, MBBS, FRACS, FAOrthA

KEYWORDS

• Knee • Osteotomies • Navigation • Advantages • Pitfalls • Techniques • Outcomes

KEY POINTS

• Computer navigation is now recognized to improve the accuracy and the precision of the correction angle in realignment osteotomies around the knee, and therefore should be considered as a useful tool.

• It allows an intraoperative assessment of limb alignment throughout the range of motion.

• By assessing the sagittal alignment, it avoids inadvertent change in the tibial posterior slope angle and it may aid complex osteotomies.

• The current limitations of computer-assisted navigation are mainly the additional time, the cost-effectiveness, and a long learning curve to avoid potential pitfalls.

• If the additional accuracy in using navigation is proved, the clinical benefits remain unclear, requiring further clinical follow-up, including a discussion related to the ideal alignment.

INTRODUCTION

Realignment osteotomies around the knee are now well-established techniques in the treatment of extraarticular deformity,[1]. They are used to treat knee osteoarthritis (OA) by shifting the lower limb mechanical axis in the coronal plane and therefore redistributing weight-bearing forces from the worn to the well-preserved compartment,[2] as well as managing joint instability in the sagittal plane.[3]

Osteotomy is a technically demanding procedure and accuracy of intraoperative correction is a key factor for achieving successful limb alignment. Surgical imprecision of only a few degrees may result in the failure of the osteotomies with poor clinical benefits.[4] In addition, a set target point for all patients is inconsistent with this bespoke

Conflict of interest: The authors declare that they have no competing interests. No benefits in any form have been received or will be received from a commercial party related directly or indirectly to the subject of this article.
Author contributions: All authors were fully involved in the study and the preparation of the article. They have read and approved the article. In addition, the article has not been published, and will not be submitted for publication, elsewhere.
Sydney Orthopaedic Research Institute (SORI), Level 1, The Gallery 445 Victoria Avenue, Chatswood, New South Wales 2067, Australia
* Corresponding author.
E-mail addresses: thomasneri@orange.fr; tneri@sori.com.au

Clin Sports Med 38 (2019) 451–469
https://doi.org/10.1016/j.csm.2019.02.009
sportsmed.theclinics.com

approach.[5] Achieving this patient-specific accuracy therefore implies 3 conditions: a reliable surgical technique with a stable fixation,[6] accurate preoperative planning of correction,[7] and a precise control of the intraoperative alignment correction.

The first condition has been better controlled since the development of reliable osteotomy techniques[8] and strong fixation ensured by a locking plate.[6]

The second condition involves preoperative measuring of limb alignment and calculation of the correction to perform during the osteotomy. With the development of computerized measurement systems and most recently three-dimensional (3D) assessment systems allowing even the measurement of the rotational component of a deformity, the preoperative planning accuracy has been improved.[9,10]

However, reaching the same level of accuracy during the procedure remains challenging, making the third condition (ie, intraoperative alignment control) essential. Historically, many techniques have been used to determine intraoperative alignment correction, such as cables, grids, and fluoroscopic confirmation. However, many limitations can occur, such as a bent cable, malalignment of guide position, suboptimal or low-quality fluoroscopy image, limb rotation, obstruction with the tourniquet in obese patients, and no sagittal assessment, and subsequently none have proved satisfactory.[7,11,12] An intraoperative error of calculating the mechanical axis can lead to inaccurate correction in the coronal plane with the risk of creating an oblique joint line, which is difficult to revise to total knee arthroplasty (TKA),[13] undercorrection or overcorrection with the risk of OA progression in the worn or contralateral compartments,[14] and an inadvertent change in the tibial posterior slope angle.[15–17] To avoid these issues, other techniques have been proposed: gap measurement,[18] patient-specific instrumentation,[19] and computer navigation, which are discussed here.

Computer navigation systems have been developed to improve both the accuracy and precision of orthopedic procedures. With these aims, this system was first developed for the spine and then for joint replacement procedures.[20] It has been shown to be effective for accurate restoration of neutral alignment in patients undergoing TKA,[21] suggesting that computer-assisted systems may be used for knee osteotomy to help surgeons to determine the intraoperative adequacy of alignment correction.[22] By providing a more precise analysis of limb alignment and a capacity to make multiplane measurements in real time, this navigation system has been increasingly used in knee osteotomies, for the proximal tibia (high tibial osteotomy [HTO])[23–28] and the distal femur (distal femoral osteotomy [DFO]).[13,29]

However, navigated surgery is time consuming with an additional cost, so justification should be sought before recommending the use of this technology.[30] Although the theoretic advantages related to the enhanced precision and accuracy have been established for HTO, it remains debatable whether these improvements lead to enhanced clinical outcomes.[31–33]

Therefore, this article provides orthopedic surgeons with a comprehensive rationale for using computer-assisted navigation in combination with knee osteotomy, with a summary of its advantages and limitations, and outlines the authors' surgical technique for navigated knee osteotomy, as well as potential pitfalls and clinical outcomes from our series.

RATIONALE AND THEORETICAL POINTS ON NAVIGATION SYSTEM
Navigation Systems

Navigation systems can broadly be divided into 2 types: image-based systems depending on either preoperative computed tomography (CT) scans or intraoperative fluoroscopy, and, more commonly, imageless systems using intraoperative data acquisition to build an anatomic model.[34] Imageless systems have become more popular because of less irradiation and reduced cost, and mostly thanks to the ability to provide real-time measurements.[34]

Briefly, the setup of navigation system requires 2 steps: instrument calibration, and femoral and tibial bony fixation of pins with markers (active or passive). After registration of anatomic landmarks and determination of hip/knee/ankle joint center, a 3D model of the lower limb is created including the coronal and the sagittal axes. Obtaining these data at the beginning, during, and at the end of surgery allows the surgeon to assess the effect of a procedure on the axis, knee laxity, and range of motion.[34]

Advantages

- The first advantage of a navigation system is to increase the accuracy and precision of the planned correction. Accuracy refers to the degree of closeness to the target angle value. Precision refers to the reliability of obtaining the planned correction and to the capacity to reduce outliers.[35] The lower incidence of instrumental errors, and the ability to calculate full anatomic and mechanical axis from the hip to the ankle, have been proved in many studies.[23–28,36] Good accuracy and precision are required to reach the ideal correction.[37] Inaccurate correction can lead to osteotomy failure. Undercorrection leads to progression of the osteoarthritis of the worn compartment and patient dissatisfaction.[38] Overcorrection can lead to patellar subluxation, patella baja,[39] joint opening, and rapid degeneration of the contralateral compartment.[40]
- Unlike conventional techniques, a navigation system allows an intraoperative assessment of limb alignment throughout the range of motion, and not just with the knee in full extension.[34] The navigated osteotomy can be individually tailored to the exact pattern of osteoarthritis or malalignment of the patient's knee in different functional positions.[5] Because much knee function occurs on a bent knee, the amount of correction in all positions can therefore be optimized.
- The third main advantage is to assess the sagittal alignment, avoiding inadvertent alteration of the tibial posterior slope angle[15–17] and aiding more complex osteotomies, such as double-level (tibia and femur) or multiplanar osteotomies for severe deformation or knee instability.[13] For medial opening wedge HTO (MOWHTO), Lustig and colleagues[15] showed there was a significant increase in bony tibial slope in both compartments following MOWHTO, and that the tibial change was larger in the medial compartment compared with the lateral compartment. Noyes and colleagues[16] reported that even a small gap error of 1 mm could result in a change of the posterior slope of approximately 2°.
- The ability to give real-time measurements provides many advantages.[34] The alignment can be carefully adjusted and, rather than using only preoperative measurements to guide the amount of correction, it quantifies the alignment change as the osteotomy is being performed. The osteotomy is only fixed in place when the precise alignment that is needed has been achieved. Soft tissue laxity can be measured and accounted for in the correction, in order to avoid overcorrection. It can also provide dynamic information on the ligament balancing (information on medial or lateral soft tissue), range of motion, postoperative fixation stability, leg axis during simulated full weight bearing, and information on the status of the cortical hinge. As explained by Song and Bae,[41] accurate control of the position of the cortical hinge and the dynamic assessment of the plastic deformation of the opposite cortex when using navigation guidance can help to avoid hinge fractures in osteotomy. Given the possibility to easily check the intraoperative alignment, navigation systems allow a reduction in the

use of fluoroscopy and therefore decreased radiation exposure, and also may compensate for the shortcomings of preoperative radiographic planning.
- In addition, navigation can be considered as a teaching tool, to explain the procedure and to shorten the learning curve, as well as a research instrument to record accurately intraoperative correction angles or kinematics.[41]

Disadvantages

The current limitations of computer navigation are the additional time, the cost-effectiveness, and the long learning curves to avoid potential pitfalls and complications.[30,35]

- Often considered by surgeons as the main limitation, use of navigation requires setup (calibration, bony fixation) and registration, leading to additional theater time from 10 to 30 minutes.[30] This longer time may be associated with an increased incidence of deep infection.[42]
- Apart from medical considerations, these high-cost technologies increase economic burden. Goradia[43] indicated that only high-volume centers can support this additional cost. Paradoxically, the navigated surgery is more beneficial for low-volume surgeons, who may have only a limited access to this technology.[25,43]
- In addition to complications related to the osteotomy procedure,[1] mainly lateral cortex or intraarticular fracture, delayed union, and loss of correction, navigation systems have to be considered as a procedure by themselves with their own complications.[30] However, specific complications of navigation are uncommon and mainly related to the use of reference array (pins), including additional incisions for insertion of pins increasing the risk of wound complications including infection,[42] iatrogenic fracture around the pins,[44] neurovascular injury during insertion of pins, and heterotopic ossification.[45] Gebhard and colleagues[25] highlighted that the complication rate is related to surgeon experience, and that navigation requires a long learning curve. Most mistakes are related to registration failures and navigation system malfunctions/misuse.[37] These potential pitfalls are discussed later.

Does Computer-assisted Navigation Osteotomy Improve Outcomes Compared with a Conventional Procedure?

Many case series of navigated HTO have shown good outcomes in terms of postoperative coronal alignment and clinical outcomes.[23–28] Results concerning tibial slope control have been conflicting, but many studies used the first version of the software, which does not allow good assessment of the sagittal alignment.[41] Our impression from these studies, which seemed to recommend the navigation procedure, was that a significant part of a patient's improvement would most likely be from the HTO, but without a comparison group this cannot be assessed. As far as the authors are aware, there are few comparative investigations of the outcome of navigated osteotomy versus conventional techniques, and closer scrutiny of the literature reveals methodological deficiencies. Among them, the main limitation is caused by a change in surgical technique over time with the use of navigation at a time when there were concurrent changes in surgical techniques and fixation methods.

Ribeiro and colleagues,[23] in a controlled clinical study, concluded that the navigation system allowed a significantly better control of tibial slope and better Lysholm score compared with a conventional HTO technique, but the conventional group was based on an older series with different plates. Recently, a retrospective study also proposed a comparison between both techniques.[46] The group comparison was not based on the time line but on the surgeon (some of them used navigation, others performed conventional HTO). The investigators concluded that navigation allowed greater success in achieving the desired correction value in the coronal plane and reduced outliers. Akamatsu and colleagues,[47] in a comparative study of HTO with and without a combined CT-based and image-free navigation system, reported that navigation restored normal coronal and sagittal plane knee joint alignment more frequently compared with a conventional technique.

In summary, as concluded by recent meta-analysis[31,33,48] and literature review,[32,41,49] navigation systems increase the accuracy and the reliability of the correction, but there is no clear evidence that this increased precision leads to better clinical outcomes or longer survivorship.

What About Distal Femoral Osteotomy?

DFO is a less common procedure that can be performed in isolation or combined with an HTO in a double-level osteotomy. Isolated DFO can be used for the correction of valgus malalignment to unload the lateral compartment without overloading the medial compartment, by restoring a neutral alignment (rather than overcorrecting as in HTO) and returning the tension side to the lateral side.[13] The double-level osteotomy is used for excessive deformities when a single osteotomy can result in an oblique joint line.

Evidence for the use of navigation in combination with DFO is limited to clinical series[13,29] without a comparative study. For double-level osteotomy, Babis and colleagues[50] reported on 29 knees, with 2 cases of undercorrection and 15 cases of overcorrection with a conventional procedure. The main difficulty is that the landmarks change after the first osteotomy, increasing the risk of malalignment with the second osteotomy. To avoid this issue, Saragaglia and colleagues[13] proposed the use of navigation. They reported 92.7% (39 of 42 knees) of limbs aligned (hip-knee-ankle [HKA] angle) with only 1 case of an oblique joint line, suggesting that computer assistance allows control of the HKA angle at every step of the procedure, making the double-level correction more precise.

PERFORMING A NAVIGATED HIGH TIBIAL OSTEOTOMY: OUR SURGICAL TECHNIQUE

As with every procedure, navigated osteotomy requires technical knowledge and a learning curve. In the following part, a detailed surgical technique of a navigated MOWHTO, based on our 10 years of experience, is presented.[15]

Preoperative Assessment

Preoperative planning is undertaken with a long-leg weight-bearing alignment film. The width of the plateau is calculated and the current mechanical axis assessed. The Fujisawa point (defined as 62% of the width measured from the medial side) is used to plan the mechanical axis.[51] These measurements are then correlated with the navigation measurements obtained intraoperatively.

Setup

A large operating room is required to set up all the equipment, including arthroscopic tower, navigation camera, navigation and osteotomy instruments, and portable fluoroscopy image intensifier C-arm. The patient is placed supine with a thigh tourniquet and a foot bolster and side support to support the knee at 90°. The authors use the Stryker Navigation System with the Precision Knee module (Stryker, Kalamazoo, MI). This system is an image-free infrared system allowing calculation of the axial, rotational, and translational positions of the tibia with respect to the femur.

Diagnostic, Therapeutic, and Registration Arthroscopy

A knee arthroscopy is first performed, for systematic examination (cartilage, menisci, cruciate ligament, synovium) of the knee and confirmation that the lateral and patellofemoral compartments are well preserved. This arthroscopy also permits treatment of any intraarticular disorder, such as associated degenerative meniscal tears.

Navigation Registration with Arthroscopic Assistance

After instrument calibration, percutaneous partially threaded 3.0-mm pins are placed into the tibial shaft and distal femur allowing the attachment of the trackers.

The center of the hip is registered by circumduction movements (**Fig. 1**A). Knee arthroscopy is then performed to register intraarticular landmarks necessary to calculate limb axis. With a pointing device introduced through the anteromedial portal, the center of the distal femur (the same point at which the intramedullary rod would be placed during TKA) and the center of the proximal tibia (tibial anterior cruciate ligament footprint) are registered (**Fig. 1**B). Surface landmarks of the knee (tibial tubercle, medial/lateral epicondyles) are then also digitized. The center of the ankle is calculated from the registration of the medial and lateral malleoli (**Fig. 1**C).

This stage completes the registration process and the software calculates the mechanical femoral and tibial axes and displays the mechanical alignment in the coronal and sagittal planes (**Fig. 2**), and this is then correlated to preoperative imaging. The ligament balancing and the range of motion are also recorded in order to check whether the postosteotomy maximal values (mainly extension) are similar to the preosteotomy value.

High Tibial Osteotomy

A 10-cm incision is made midway between the tibial tubercle and the posteromedial tibial cortex, beginning 1 cm inferior to the joint line and extending distally. The sartorius fascia is sharply divided in line with the skin incision followed by posterior reflection of sartorius, gracilis, semitendinosus, and the superficial medial collateral ligament with its underlying periosteal attachment. The patellar tendon and retropatellar bursa are exposed anteriorly and protected. This exposure achieves a subperiosteal exposure of the proposed site for the osteotomy. Under fluoroscopy, a 2-mm guide pin is advanced from the medial side crossing obliquely above the tibial tuberosity and toward the tip of the fibula, sitting 15 mm distal to the lateral tibial plateau to prevent the osteotomy from disrupting the joint. The osteotomy follows immediately distal to the guide pin to center the hinge of the osteotomy at the proximal tibiofibular joint. The osteotomy is performed under fluoroscopy using an oscillating saw for the

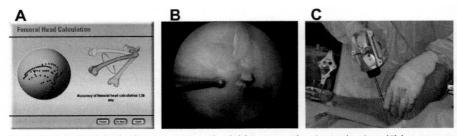

Fig. 1. Determining limb alignment using the (*A*) hip center by circumduction, (*B*) knee center with a pointing device registering arthroscopically, and (*C*) ankle center using surface malleoli landmarks.

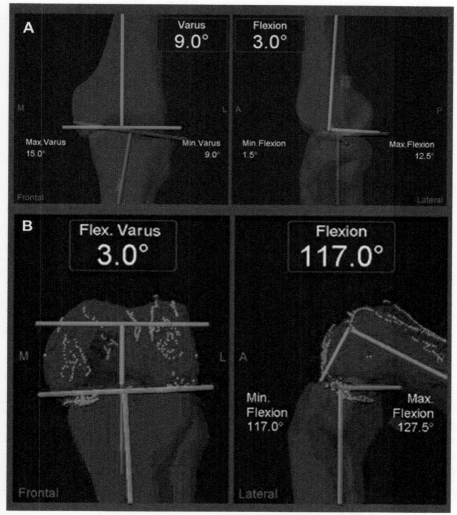

Fig. 2. Intraoperative assessment of the malalignment in coronal and sagittal planes (*A*) in extension and (*B*) throughout the range of motion.

outer medial and anterior cortices and completed with flexible osteotomes, carried to within 5 mm of the lateral cortex.

Navigated Opening and Osteotomy Fixation

A laminar spreader is placed posteriorly and the osteotomy opened until the desired alignment of mechanical valgus in full extension is achieved. The posterior opening is measured and checked to be in line with preoperative calculations, after which a locking plate is secured in place with 3 to 4 screws proximally and 3 to 4 distally, taking care to hold the knee aligned in both planes, confirmed with navigation. Maintenance of tibial slope is confirmed by ensuring that full extension, as measured precorrection, is maintained. A wedge of femoral head allograft is placed into the osteotomy gap and then impacted. The gap filling and the osteotomy stability are checked by fluoroscopy.

Final alignment is checked and recorded, analyzing the coronal and the sagittal alignment (**Fig. 3**).

Postoperative Plan Regimen

The postoperative rehabilitation program includes a 4-week period of touch weight bearing with a knee brace set from 0° to 90° of flexion, followed by 4 weeks of gradual progression to full weight bearing with brace off.

Potential Navigation Pitfalls

Surgeons have to be aware of potential pitfalls, such as registration failures, line-of-sight issues, and mechanical or software malfunctions.[41] Surgeons therefore have to be comfortable with conventional techniques, in case such issues with the navigation system occur intraoperatively.

- Mechanical axis and angle value are calculated from registered landmarks. If the landmarks are not accurately registered, the computer cannot compensate for this.[25,52] This limitation should be considered, because the navigation system cannot identify features that the surgeon cannot define. A check comparing initial intraoperative data (coronal and sagittal angles, maximal flexion and extension values) and the preoperative calculations is necessary.
- Leading to the same inaccuracy, pins have to be securely fixed. If there is movement of the trackers, all measurements may be inaccurate. To avoid this issue, bicortical fixation in the metaphyseal areas is recommended.[44]
- For navigation systems using passive reflective markers, surgeons need to avoid contamination with blood, which can block reflection and transmission.
- Aside from technical pitfalls, measurements errors caused by computer, camera, or trackers can occur.[41,52] With the new navigation systems, these errors are less than 1 mm.[41,52]

The authors recommend also to check every value displayed on the computer to track mistakes. Navigation is an accurate and helpful tool but cannot be considered to be foolproof technology. A comparison with the initial intraoperative data (coronal and sagittal angles, maximal flexion and extension values) and the preoperative data is necessary.

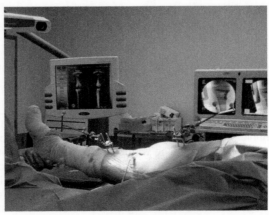

Fig. 3. Intraoperative view of the final alignment check after a navigated MOWHTO.

- For the coronal limb alignment, there is a potential discrepancy between the non-weight-bearing navigated value of preosteotomy alignment and standing loaded radiographic preoperative value.[53] Yaffe and colleagues[54] reported a difference of 8° between navigated and radiographic measurement values. To avoid these pitfalls, surgeons can simulate weight bearing by applying a varus external force during the registration step until the navigated value of the preoperative alignment matches the radiographic value. The authors also recommend checking the dynamic range of coronal alignment under applied varus and valgus force before performing the osteotomy. For the amount of correction, a double check with the preoperative plan is also recommended.[53] Preoperative templating is mandatory should intraoperative navigation fail.
- Navigation allows assessment of alignment with increasing knee flexion, which is particularly relevant to more posterior wear patterns, and should be taken into account when planning the desired correction.
- For the sagittal alignment, the postosteotomy maximal degree of extension should match the preosteotomy value.[15] If it is increased, the tibial slope has most likely been increased and the correction should be reevaluated.

OUR CLINICAL EXPERIENCE WITH NAVIGATED HIGH TIBIAL OSTEOTOMY
Objective

To compare radiographic and clinical functional outcomes between patients treated with navigated knee osteotomy and those treated through a conventional procedure.

Method

From our prospective database, we identified all patients treated for osteotomy around the knee by 3 surgeons, between November 2002 and September 2018 (**Fig. 4**). From this consecutive cohort, we included only patients having the 2 main osteotomy procedures: medial opening wedge HTO (MOWHTO) to treat varus malalignment and lateral opening wedge DFO (LOWDFO) to treat valgus malalignment. Patients having other osteotomy procedures were excluded. MOWHTO and LOWDFO patients were divided into 2 subgroups: navigated osteotomy (all patients after

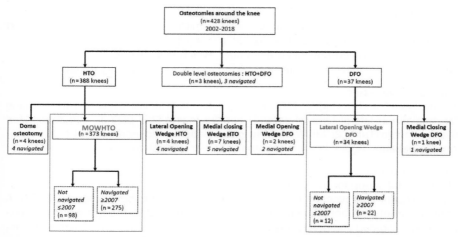

Fig. 4. Recruitment. From the consecutive cohort of knee osteotomies, only patients with MOWHTO and lateral opening wedge DFO procedures have been assessed.

January 2008 and some patients between May 2007 and December 2007) or nonnavigated osteotomy. Inclusion criteria were the following: (1) MOWHTO and LOWDFO procedures performed in our department, (2) for osteoarthritis or knee instability, (3) with a minimum of 1-year follow-up. Patients who had (1) a previous knee osteotomy (2), knee osteotomy associated with a knee arthroplasty, or (3) active psychosis/ significant mental disability were excluded. Based on these criteria, 373 knees (333 patients) were included in the MOWHTO groups (98 nonnavigated and 275 navigated) and 34 knees (32 patients) were included in the LOWDFO groups (12 nonnavigated and 22 navigated).

To ensure comparable groups, demographics (gender, age, body mass index) and knee side were collected. Clinical scores, including the International Knee Documentation Committee (IKDC)[55] subjective knee evaluation form, the Knee injury and Osteoarthritis Outcome Scores (KOOS),[56] and the Western Ontario and McMaster Universities (WOMAC) Osteoarthritis Index[57] were collected preoperatively and at last follow-up (at least 12 months after surgery). Preoperative and postoperative long-leg standing alignment films were analyzed to assess the extent of preoperative coronal deformity (HKA angle), and the postsurgical correction achieved compared with the predetermined target angle (182° for valgizing, and 178° for varizing surgery). Meniscal and cartilage status, using the International Cartilage Repair Society (ICRS) scores[58] were analyzed at the time of surgery. Treatment details, such as procedure used, duration of surgery, and fixation plates used, were also reported. Any complications and reoperations were recorded.

All statistical analyses were performed using SPSS Statistics software (version 21, SPSS Inc., Chicago, IL) and the significance threshold was set at $P<.05$. Quantitative data are expressed as the mean plus or minus standard deviation (minimum, maximum). For comparison of quantitative parameters, Student t test was used if a normal distribution hypothesis was confirmed. Otherwise, the nonparametric Mann-Whitney test was used. For comparison of qualitative parameters, the χ^2 test was used if a normal distribution hypothesis was confirmed. Otherwise, the Fisher exact test were used. For clinical scores, the change has been analyzed relative to the preoperative value.

Results

Patient demographics
Nonnavigated and navigated groups were similar regarding demographics and causes (**Table 1**), except for the age at surgery between LOWDFO procedures. Because nonnavigated patients are younger, which is known to be associated with improved results, this issue would not be in favor of the superiority of navigation.

Intraoperative results
Nonnavigated and navigated MOWHTO groups were similar regarding ICRS grade for medial and lateral femoral condyle and for lateral tibia plateau and associated meniscal tears (**Table 2**). MOWHTO-navigated patients had more grade 4 than nonnavigated patients. Again, this issue would not favor navigation.

Functional scores
The mean follow-up for the scores was 1.76 ± 1.72 years.[1,15]

A significant improvement in clinical scores was found in both groups ($P<.001$). A comparison of the improvement in clinical scores related to the preoperative value between navigated and nonnavigated groups for both procedures revealed no statistically significant difference for IKDC, KOOS (pain, activity of daily living, sports, quality of life) and WOMAC scores (pain, stiffness, function, and total) (**Fig. 5**). Only the

Table 1
Comparison between navigated and nonnavigated groups for demographic data and causes

Group	BMI		Gender, M/F (n)		Age at Surgery (y)		Knee Side, R/L (n)		Cause, OA/Instability (n)	
MOWHTO										
Nonnavigated	28.7 ± 4.4 (21, 41)	P = .620	86/12	P = .054	48.2 ± 11.3 (19, 69)	P = .994	50/48	P = .528	93/5	P = .664
Navigated	29.7 ± 6.1 (19, 59)		215/61		48.5 ± 8 (25, 65)		151/125		267/9	
All	29.4 ± 5.6 (19, 59)	—	301/73	—	48.4 ± 9 (19, 69)	—	201/173	—	360/14	—
LOWDFO										
Nonnavigated	26.4 ± 4.2 (18, 32)	P = .764	9/3	P = .258	30.6 ± 11.7 (16, 50)	P = .001[a]	8/4	P = .503	12/0	—
Navigated	28.9 ± 5.1 (21.9, 38)		12/10		43.2 ± 6.3 (30, 53)		12/10		22/0	—
All	27.6 ± 4.7 (18, 38)	—	21/13	—	38.7 ± 10.4 (16, 53)	—	20/14	—	34/0	—

Abbreviations: F, female; L, left; M, male; R, right.
[a] P<.05.

Table 2
Comparison between navigated and nonnavigated groups for intraoperative findings and associated cartilage procedures

| Group | ICRS Grading (%) | | | | Cartilage Procedure (n) | | Meniscal Lesions (n) |
| | Normal/Grade 1/Grade 2/Grade 3/Grade 4 | | | | Debridement/Microfracture/MACI | | |
	Medial Femoral Condyle	Medial Tibia Plateau	Lateral Femoral Condyle	Lateral Tibia Plateau	Medial Compartment	Lateral Compartment	Medial/Lateral
MOWHTO							
Nonnavigated	3/3/7/31/55 $P = .113$	7/14/24/21/34 $P = .004$[a]	62/21/10/0/7 $P = .083$	41/55/3/0/0 $P = .213$	NA	NA	15/4 $P = .177$
Navigated	5/2/4/19/71	5/4/15/15/62	58/26/12/2/2	36/46/16/2/0	4/26/7	1/0/0	68/7
LOWDFO							
Nonnavigated	NA —	NA	NA —	NA	NA	NA	0/0 —
Navigated	38/38/25/0/0	63/25/13/0/0	13/0/0/25/63	13/0/0/13/75	1/0/0	0/1/0	0/6

Abbreviations: MACI, matrix-induced autologous chondrocyte implant; NA, not available.
[a] $P<.05$.

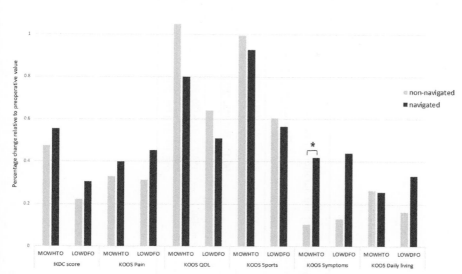

Fig. 5. Comparison of change in functional scores over time for IKDC subjective and KOOS subscales scores related to the preoperative value between navigated and nonnavigated groups. ADL, activities of daily living; QOL, quality of life. * = P<.05.

MOWHTO-navigated patients showed greater improvement in the symptoms subscale of KOOS compared with the nonnavigated patients (P<.001).

Alignment and duration of surgery
Navigated and nonnavigated groups of both procedures were comparable for preoperative alignment (**Table 3**). Use of navigation in MOWHTO resulted in postoperative coronal alignment closer to the target angle (mean, 182.8°) compared with nonnavigated MOWHTO procedures, which led to an average overcorrection (mean, 184.4°) (P = .001). No significant difference was observed with the DFO procedure. Use of navigation increased duration of surgery for MOWHTO (P = .001), but not for LOWDFO.

Complications
All complications are reported in **Table 4**. Use of navigation did not change the complication rate between HTO and DFO procedures.

Discussion
Use of navigation had additional questionable clinical benefit in self-reported symptoms when used in combination with MOWHTO. It did not improve the other clinical functional scores. Regarding the precision of alignment correction, computer-assisted surgery resulted in an outcome closer to the targeted angular correction. These findings are in line with current literature, by concluding that navigation is a useful tool to control the intraoperative alignment correction, possibly more for inexperienced or low-volume surgeons, but without a clear clinical benefit.

However, several limitations should be noted. First, the comparison of navigated and nonnavigated groups is biased because of a change in surgical technique over time with the use of new fixation methods, such as locking plates. Second, the DFO group included only a small number of patients, leading to a lack of power. Third,

Table 3
Comparison between navigated and nonnavigated groups for preoperative and postoperative alignment and duration of surgery

Group	Preoperative HKA (°)		Postoperative HKA (°)		Duration of Surgery (min)	
MOWHTO						
Nonnavigated	174.7 ± 2.5 (172, 177)	P = .610	184.4 ± 2.3 (180, 190)	P = .001[a]	84.3 ± 23.5 (45, 150)	P = .001[a]
Navigated	173.8 ± 2.7 (166, 179)		182.8 ± 1.7 (180, 190)		97.1 ± 27.5 (55, 180)	
All	173.9 ± 2.7 (166, 179)	—	183 ± 1.8 (180, 190)	—	90.1 ± 26.1 (45, 180)	—
LOWDFO						
Nonnavigated	185.9 ± 2.2 (182, 190)	P = .574	177.3 ± 1.6 (175, 180)	P = .490	114.7 ± 37.9 (80, 210)	P = .542
Navigated	186.5 ± 2.4 (182, 191)		177.7 ± 1.1 (176, 180)		115.4 ± 23.3 (75, 160)	
All	186.1 ± 2.3 (182, 191)	—	177.6 ± 1.3 (175, 180)	—	115.1 ± 31.4 (75, 210)	—

[a] P<.05.

Table 4
Complications

Group	Hardware Removal: n (%)	OA Progression Requiring a Conversion to TKA: n (%)	Delayed Union: n (%)	Nonunion Requiring a Revision Surgery: n (%)	Iterative Arthroscopy for Meniscectomy: n (%)	Wound Hematoma: n (%)
			Complications n= (%)			
MOWHTO						
Nonnavigated	20 (20.4)	2 (2)	0	0	1 (1)	1 (1)
Navigated	38 (13.8)	0	2 (0.7)	2 (0.7)	2 (0.7)	1 (0.4)
All	58 (15.5)	2 (1)	2 (0.5)	2 (0.5)	3 (0.8)	2 (0.5)
LOWDFO						
Nonnavigated	2 (16.7)	1 (8.3)	1 (8.3)	0	0	0
Navigated	5 (22.7)	0	0	1 (4.5)	0	0
All	7 (20.6)	1 (2.9)	1 (2.9)	1 (2.9)	0	0

with a mean clinical follow-up of 1.76 years, our study cannot foresee the longer-term influence of navigation.

SUMMARY

Despite encouraging results for the use of navigation in knee osteotomies, some questions are still unresolved.

- The definition of the ideal alignment in the coronal, sagittal, and axial planes is necessary to determine the target angular correction. Navigation is a tool allowing a more precise osteotomy but does not provide all the information required to restore physiologic alignment and kinematics. Biomechanical studies are required to define ideal alignments in each plane to provide individualized optimal conditions for articular cartilage health and ligament stability.
- This intraoperative guide only allows simulated weight-bearing assessment of limb alignment. Further studies analyzing the relationship between supine alignment, simulated weight bearing with navigation, and dynamic full weight-bearing are needed.
- Computer-assisted surgery remains an added cost, and is mainly available in high-volume centers, although it may be more beneficial for low-volume surgeons. Reduced price and increased availability are therefore necessary.
- In order to decrease the long learning curve and the potential pitfalls, new software that is easier and simpler needs to be developed.
- To answer the question of whether more accurate correction leads to improved clinical outcomes and longer survivorship, randomized or at least controlled trials with long follow-up are necessary.

To summarize, navigation represents an accurate and reliable tool for surgeons performing knee osteotomy for OA and ligament instability. This technique provides intraoperative real-time guidance of the degree of correction for coronal and sagittal alignment throughout the range of motion. The accuracy and the precision of the final correction angle in realignment osteotomies provided by computer-assisted surgery is now well recognized in the literature and also by our results. However, the clinical benefits remain unclear, requiring further clinical follow-up, including an ongoing discussion related to the ideal alignment and more dynamic assessment.

REFERENCES

1. Amendola A, Bonasia DE. Results of high tibial osteotomy: review of the literature. Int Orthop 2010;34(2):155–60.
2. Coventry MB. Osteotomy of the upper portion of the tibia for degenerative arthritis of the knee. a preliminary report. J Bone Joint Surg Am 1965;47:984–90.
3. Noyes FR, Barber-Westin SD, Hewett TE. High tibial osteotomy and ligament reconstruction for varus angulated anterior cruciate ligament-deficient knees. Am J Sports Med 2000;28(3):282–96.
4. Sharma L, Song J, Felson DT, et al. The role of knee alignment in disease progression and functional decline in knee osteoarthritis. JAMA 2001;286(2):188–95.
5. Feucht MJ, Minzlaff P, Saier T, et al. Degree of axis correction in valgus high tibial osteotomy: proposal of an individualised approach. Int Orthop 2014;38(11): 2273–80.
6. Staubli AE, De Simoni C, Babst R, et al. TomoFix: a new LCP-concept for open wedge osteotomy of the medial proximal tibia–early results in 92 cases. Injury 2003;34(Suppl 2):B55–62.
7. Dugdale TW, Noyes FR, Styer D. Preoperative planning for high tibial osteotomy. The effect of lateral tibiofemoral separation and tibiofemoral length. Clin Orthop 1992;274:248–64.
8. Lobenhoffer P, Agneskirchner JD. Improvements in surgical technique of valgus high tibial osteotomy. Knee Surg Sports Traumatol Arthrosc 2003;11(3):132–8.
9. Schröter S, Ihle C, Mueller J, et al. Digital planning of high tibial osteotomy. Inter-rater reliability by using two different software. Knee Surg Sports Traumatol Arthrosc 2013;21(1):189–96.
10. Sailhan F, Jacob L, Hamadouche M. Differences in limb alignment and femoral mechanical-anatomical angles using two dimension versus three dimension radiographic imaging. Int Orthop 2017;41(10):2009–16.
11. Krettek C, Miclau T, Grün O, et al. Intraoperative control of axes, rotation and length in femoral and tibial fractures. Technical note. Injury 1998;29(Suppl 3): C29–39.
12. Saleh M, Harriman P, Edwards DJ. A radiological method for producing precise limb alignment. J Bone Joint Surg Br 1991;73(3):515–6.
13. Saragaglia D, Chedal-Bornu B, Rouchy RC, et al. Role of computer-assisted surgery in osteotomies around the knee. Knee Surg Sports Traumatol Arthrosc 2016; 24(11):3387–95.
14. Cerejo R, Dunlop DD, Cahue S, et al. The influence of alignment on risk of knee osteoarthritis progression according to baseline stage of disease. Arthritis Rheum 2002;46(10):2632–6.
15. Lustig S, Scholes CJ, Costa AJ, et al. Different changes in slope between the medial and lateral tibial plateau after open-wedge high tibial osteotomy. Knee Surg Sports Traumatol Arthrosc 2013;21(1):32–8.
16. Noyes FR, Goebel SX, West J. Opening wedge tibial osteotomy: the 3-triangle method to correct axial alignment and tibial slope. Am J Sports Med 2005; 33(3):378–87.
17. Bae DK, Ko YW, Kim SJ, et al. Computer-assisted navigation decreases the change in the tibial posterior slope angle after closed-wedge high tibial osteotomy. Knee Surg Sports Traumatol Arthrosc 2016;24(11):3433–40.

18. Schröter S, Ihle C, Elson DW, et al. Surgical accuracy in high tibial osteotomy: coronal equivalence of computer navigation and gap measurement. Knee Surg Sports Traumatol Arthrosc 2016;24(11):3410–7.
19. Donnez M, Ollivier M, Munier M, et al. Are three-dimensional patient-specific cutting guides for open wedge high tibial osteotomy accurate? An in vitro study. J Orthop Surg 2018;13(1):171.
20. Delp SL, Stulberg SD, Davies B, et al. Computer assisted knee replacement. Clin Orthop Relat Res 1998;(354):49–56.
21. Petursson G, Fenstad AM, Gøthesen Ø, et al. Computer-assisted compared with conventional total knee replacement: a multicenter parallel-group randomized controlled trial. J Bone Joint Surg Am 2018;100(15):1265–74.
22. Lee D-H, Nha K-W, Park S-J, et al. Preoperative and postoperative comparisons of navigation and radiologic limb alignment measurements after high tibial osteotomy. Arthroscopy 2012;28(12):1842–50.
23. Ribeiro CH, Severino NR, Moraes de Barros Fucs PM. Opening wedge high tibial osteotomy: navigation system compared to the conventional technique in a controlled clinical study. Int Orthop 2014;38(8):1627–31.
24. Akamatsu Y, Mitsugi N, Mochida Y, et al. Navigated opening wedge high tibial osteotomy improves intraoperative correction angle compared with conventional method. Knee Surg Sports Traumatol Arthrosc 2012;20(3):586–93.
25. Gebhard F, Krettek C, Hüfner T, et al. Reliability of computer-assisted surgery as an intraoperative ruler in navigated high tibial osteotomy. Arch Orthop Trauma Surg 2011;131(3):297–302.
26. Heijens E, Kornherr P, Meister C. The role of navigation in high tibial osteotomy: a study of 50 patients. Orthopedics 2009;32(10 Suppl):40–3.
27. Iorio R, Vadalà A, Giannetti S, et al. Computer-assisted high tibial osteotomy: preliminary results. Orthopedics 2010;33(10 Suppl):82–6.
28. Reising K, Strohm PC, Hauschild O, et al. Computer-assisted navigation for the intraoperative assessment of lower limb alignment in high tibial osteotomy can avoid outliers compared with the conventional technique. Knee Surg Sports Traumatol Arthrosc 2013;21(1):181–8.
29. Saragaglia D, Mercier N, Colle P-E. Computer-assisted osteotomies for genu varum deformity: which osteotomy for which varus? Int Orthop 2010;34(2):185–90.
30. Hankemeier S, Hufner T, Wang G, et al. Navigated open-wedge high tibial osteotomy: advantages and disadvantages compared to the conventional technique in a cadaver study. Knee Surg Sports Traumatol Arthrosc 2006;14(10):917–21.
31. Wu Z-P, Zhang P, Bai J-Z, et al. Comparison of navigated and conventional high tibial osteotomy for the treatment of osteoarthritic knees with varus deformity: a meta-analysis. Int J Surg 2018;55:211–9.
32. Yan J, Musahl V, Kay J, et al. Outcome reporting following navigated high tibial osteotomy of the knee: a systematic review. Knee Surg Sports Traumatol Arthrosc 2016;24(11):3529–55.
33. Kim HJ, Yoon J-R, Choi GW, et al. Imageless navigation versus conventional open wedge high tibial osteotomy: a meta-analysis of comparative studies. Knee Surg Relat Res 2016;28(1):16–26.
34. Matsumoto T, Nakano N, Lawrence JE, et al. Current concepts and future perspectives in computer-assisted navigated total knee replacement. Int Orthop 2018. [Epub ahead of print].
35. Young SW, Safran MR, Clatworthy M. Applications of computer navigation in sports medicine knee surgery: an evidence-based review. Curr Rev Musculoskelet Med 2013;6(2):150–7.

36. Lo WN, Cheung KW, Yung SH, et al. Arthroscopy-assisted computer navigation in high tibial osteotomy for varus knee deformity. J Orthop Surg (Hong Kong) 2009; 17(1):51–5.

37. Picardo NE, Khan W, Johnstone D. Computer-assisted navigation in high tibial osteotomy: a systematic review of the literature. Open Orthop J 2012;6:305–12.

38. Ribeiro CH, Severino NR, Fucs PM. Preoperative surgical planning versus navigation system in valgus tibial osteotomy: a cross-sectional study. Int Orthop 2013;37(8):1483–6.

39. Dowd GSE, Somayaji HS, Uthukuri M. High tibial osteotomy for medial compartment osteoarthritis. Knee 2006;13(2):87–92.

40. Sim JA, Kwak JH, Yang SH, et al. Effect of weight-bearing on the alignment after open wedge high tibial osteotomy. Knee Surg Sports Traumatol Arthrosc 2010; 18(7):874–8.

41. Song SJ, Bae DK. Computer-assisted navigation in high tibial osteotomy. Clin Orthop Surg 2016;8(4):349–57.

42. Iorio R, Pagnottelli M, Vadalà A, et al. Open-wedge high tibial osteotomy: comparison between manual and computer-assisted techniques. Knee Surg Sports Traumatol Arthrosc 2013;21(1):113–9.

43. Goradia VK. Computer-assisted and robotic surgery in orthopedics: where we are in 2014. Sports Med Arthrosc Rev 2014;22(4):202–5.

44. Bonutti P, Dethmers D, Stiehl JB. Case report. Clin Orthop 2008;466(6):1499–502.

45. Citak M, Kendoff D, O'Loughlin PF, et al. Heterotopic ossification post navigated high tibial osteotomy. Knee Surg Sports Traumatol Arthrosc 2009;17(4):352–5.

46. Chang J, Scallon G, Beckert M, et al. Comparing the accuracy of high tibial osteotomies between computer navigation and conventional methods. Comput Assist Surg (Abingdon) 2017;22(1):1–8.

47. Akamatsu Y, Kobayashi H, Kusayama Y, et al. Comparative study of opening-wedge high tibial osteotomy with and without a combined computed tomography-based and image-free navigation system. Arthroscopy 2016;32(10):2072–81.

48. Han S-B, Kim HJ, Lee D-H. Effect of computer navigation on accuracy and reliability of limb alignment correction following open-wedge high tibial osteotomy: a meta-analysis. Biomed Res Int 2017;2017:3803457.

49. Hasan K, Rahman QA, Zalzal P. Navigation versus conventional high tibial osteotomy: systematic review. Springerplus 2015;4(1):271.

50. Babis GC, An K-N, Chao EYS, et al. Double level osteotomy of the knee: a method to retain joint-line obliquity. Clinical results. J Bone Joint Surg Am 2002;84-A(8): 1380–8.

51. Fujisawa Y, Masuhara K, Shiomi S. The effect of high tibial osteotomy on osteoarthritis of the knee. An arthroscopic study of 54 knee joints. Orthop Clin North Am 1979;10(3):585–608.

52. Khadem R, Yeh CC, Sadeghi-Tehrani M, et al. Comparative tracking error analysis of five different optical tracking systems. Comput Aided Surg 2000;5(2):98–107.

53. Kyung BS, Kim JG, Jang K-M, et al. Are navigation systems accurate enough to predict the correction angle during high tibial osteotomy? Comparison of navigation systems with 3-dimensional computed tomography and standing radiographs. Am J Sports Med 2013;41(10):2368–74.

54. Yaffe MA, Koo SS, Stulberg SD. Radiographic and navigation measurements of TKA limb alignment do not correlate. Clin Orthop 2008;466(11):2736–44.

55. Anderson AF, Irrgang JJ, Kocher MS, et al, International Knee Documentation Committee. The International Knee Documentation Committee Subjective Knee Evaluation Form: normative data. Am J Sports Med 2006;34(1):128–35.

56. Roos EM, Lohmander LS. The Knee injury and Osteoarthritis Outcome Score (KOOS): from joint injury to osteoarthritis. Health Qual Life Outcomes 2003;1:64.
57. Bellamy N, Buchanan WW, Goldsmith CH, et al. Validation study of WOMAC: a health status instrument for measuring clinically important patient relevant outcomes to antirheumatic drug therapy in patients with osteoarthritis of the hip or knee. J Rheumatol 1988;15(12):1833–40.
58. Brittberg M, Winalski CS. Evaluation of cartilage injuries and repair. J Bone Joint Surg Am 2003;85-A(Suppl 2):58–69.

Degenerative Meniscal Tears and High Tibial Osteotomy

Do Current Treatment Algorithms Need to Be Realigned?

Codie A. Primeau, MSc[a,b,c], Trevor B. Birmingham, PT, PhD[a,b,c],
Kristyn M. Leitch, PhD[a,b], C. Thomas Appleton, MD, PhD[b,d],
J. Robert Giffin, MD, FRCSC, MBA[a,b,c,e,f,*]

KEYWORDS

- Degenerative meniscal tear • Knee osteoarthritis • Varus gonarthrosis • Osteotomy
- Limb realignment • Prevention • Treatment algorithms

KEY POINTS

- Recurring medial knee symptoms in the presence of varus alignment and a degenerative medial meniscal tear signify medial compartment overload and early knee osteoarthritis (OA) even if joint damage is not evident on plain knee radiographs.
- Arthroscopic partial medial meniscectomy is routinely performed for these patients in areas around the world, but does not address the underlying biomechanical problem.
- As varus alignment is a strong risk factor for medial joint degeneration, we propose limb realignment surgery should be considered earlier in the treatment algorithm at a time when biomechanical intervention is more likely to modify disease.
- The rationale and low-level proof of principle exist to encourage future investigations, including randomized trials, to evaluate HTO as a disease-modifying intervention in early knee OA.

Disclosures: The authors have no disclosures to declare related to this work.
[a] Wolf Orthopaedic Biomechanics Laboratory, Fowler Kennedy Sport Medicine Clinic, University of Western Ontario, 3M Centre, Room 1220, London, Ontario N6A 3K7, Canada; [b] Bone and Joint Institute, University of Western Ontario, London Health Sciences Centre, University Hospital B6-200, London, Ontario N6A 5B5, Canada; [c] School of Physical Therapy, Faculty of Health Sciences, University of Western Ontario, 1201 Western Road, London, Ontario N6G 1H1, Canada; [d] Department of Physiology and Pharmacology, Schulich School of Medicine and Dentistry, University of Western Ontario, 1151 Richmond Street, London, Ontario N6A 5C1, Canada; [e] Department of Surgery, Schulich School of Medicine and Dentistry, University of Ontario, St. Joseph's Healthcare London, 268 Grosvenor Street, London, Ontario N6A 4V2, Canada; [f] Orthopaedic Surgery, University of Western Ontario, London, Ontario N6A 3K7, Canada
* Corresponding author. Wolf Orthopaedic Biomechanics Laboratory, Fowler Kennedy Sport Medicine Clinic, University of Western Ontario, 3M Centre, Room 1220, London, Ontario N6A 3K7, Canada.
E-mail address: rgiffin@uwo.ca

Clin Sports Med 38 (2019) 471–482
https://doi.org/10.1016/j.csm.2019.02.010
0278-5919/19/Crown Copyright © 2019 Published by Elsevier Inc. All rights reserved.

INTRODUCTION

Knee osteoarthritis (OA) is the most common chronic joint disease, affecting all joint tissues and structures by the time the disease is well established. Degenerative meniscal tears frequently appear before changes occur in the articular cartilage and subchondral bone, and should be considered early knee OA.[1–3]

A strong body of evidence suggests that varus alignment increases the risk for degenerative meniscal tears[4–7] and radiographic knee OA.[8–11] Despite the long history of limb realignment procedures, varus alignment is seldom considered to be a modifiable risk factor in knee OA by many health care providers, including orthopedic surgeons. Moreover, surgical realignment procedures that could address the underlying varus alignment, such as high tibial osteotomy (HTO), are rarely considered until much later in the course of the disease, after substantial degenerative changes have occurred and are clearly evident on plain radiographs.

The purpose of this article was to propose that medial-opening wedge HTO be considered as a treatment option for secondary prevention in patients with frequent knee symptoms, varus alignment, and degenerative meniscal tears, in the absence of radiographic OA. We provide rationale and low-level proof of principle using specific case examples. Last, we discuss caveats and challenges, along with proposed future directions for research in the area.

DEGENERATIVE MENISCAL TEARS

The menisci are fibrocartilaginous structures in the tibiofemoral joint that are vital for dynamic joint stability and load transfer. Repetitive trauma and excess loading to the knee can disrupt mechanical and biological processes, leading to meniscal degeneration, and jeopardizing the protective functions of the menisci for the joint. Degenerative meniscal tears often involve horizontal cleavage of the meniscus in middle-aged or older persons. These lesions are particularly common in persons *(with or without symptoms)* older than 50.[2,12] Although degenerative meniscal tears often exist without symptoms, many patients do seek care for episodic knee pain, catching, synovitis, effusions, and disability *(ie, symptoms of knee OA)*. Indeed, the symptoms attributed to degenerative meniscal tears may be the first indications that the OA disease process has begun to alter knee joint structures. Furthermore, numerous studies suggest meniscal pathology is associated with an increased risk for further knee joint degeneration evident on plain radiographs *(ie, incident radiographic knee OA)*.[13–18] Given the tremendous burden of knee OA and the high prevalence of degenerative meniscal tears, we believe it is crucial to explore potential disease-modifying interventions for these patients.

LOWER LIMB ALIGNMENT AND GAIT BIOMECHANICS

Numerous observational cohort studies demonstrate that varus alignment is a potent predictor of OA in the medial knee compartment, including meniscal pathology,[4–7] and incident[8,11] and progressive[5,8–11] tibiofemoral joint degeneration. For example, evidence has existed for almost 20 years that varus alignment results in a fourfold increased risk of progression in medial radiographic knee OA over as little as 18 months (adjusted odds ratio [OR] 4.09, 95% confidence interval [CI] 2.20–7.62).[10] More recently, MRI studies suggest that knees with varus alignment are twice as likely to develop medial meniscal pathology *(ie, tear, destruction, or maceration)* within 30 months compared with knees without varus alignment (adjusted OR 2.00, 95% CI 1.18, 3.40).[6] In addition, varus alignment is associated with almost 4 times the risk of developing medial articular cartilage damage in the tibiofemoral joint, evident through MRI (adjusted OR 3.59, 95% CI 1.59–8.10).[5] Several studies also show that varus alignment is associated with high rates of developing symptomatic and radiographic knee OA.[8,11] Therefore, the depth of evidence suggests varus alignment can play a critical role in both the onset and progression of medial knee OA.

Biomechanical studies also demonstrate the potent effects of lower limb alignment. Gait studies, including instrumented knee implant[19] and motion capture[20] data, show that even small changes in frontal plane alignment cause substantial shifts in the mediolateral distribution of load on the knee during walking. Most commonly quantified as the external knee adduction moment, increased medial loading during walking is positively associated with varus alignment[19,21,22] and structural OA progression.[23–26] In addition, the presence of a varus thrust (ie, bowing out of knee during gait), seen in many patients with varus alignment, is associated with increased risk of OA progression.[27–29]

CURRENT MANAGEMENT FOR DEGENERATIVE MENISCAL TEAR

Current guidelines for treatment of knee OA suggest exhausting all nonoperative forms of treatment (eg, topical or oral analgesics, physiotherapy, lifestyle modification including regular exercise and weight reduction, intra-articular corticosteroid, braces, and orthotics) before considering surgery.[30,31] Generally, clinicians will wait until a patient presents with definitive radiographic knee OA (ie, KL$\geq$2 and American College of Rheumatology Classification Criteria fulfilled) before realignment surgery is even considered as a viable treatment option. However, there is a growing body of literature that contends the disease process is well-advanced before signs of joint damage on radiographs.[32–34] It therefore stands to reason that if pre-radiographic OA can be identified by the existence of a symptomatic degenerative meniscal tear, then interventions should be started. These should include nonoperative treatments intended to alter disease progression, such as diet (ie, weight loss) and exercise, understanding that their effects can be difficult to sustain over time and knee joint degeneration may continue. Importantly, this may be particularly true in patients with varus alignment and a degenerative meniscal tear who are at increased risk of OA progression.

Arthroscopic partial meniscectomy has long been considered the treatment of choice for symptomatic degenerative meniscal tears by surgeons around the globe.[35–37] However, the continued use of this procedure for the treatment of degenerative meniscal tears (with[38–43] or without[44–47] radiographic knee OA) is not supported by a large, well-established body of evidence from numerous high-quality randomized trials, including sham-controlled[42,45,46] and comparative effectiveness studies.[38–41,43,44,47] For degenerative medial meniscal tears (DMMTs) in the presence of varus alignment, we suggest arthroscopic treatment is directed at excising torn meniscal tissue without addressing the surrounding joint environment, nor the fundamental risk factors for persistent disease activity, which evidently include biomechanical drivers such as varus alignment.

HIGH TIBIAL OSTEOTOMY

Although varus alignment is consistently identified in prospective studies to be a strong predictor of medial knee OA progression, it is seldom considered a modifiable risk factor. Medial-opening wedge HTO corrects varus alignment to reduce aberrant loading of the medial tibiofemoral compartment. Gait studies evaluating medial-opening or lateral-closing wedge HTO suggest the procedure can produce long-term (ie, 5 years) and large (ie, 50%) reductions in the magnitude of the peak knee adduction moment, a proxy measure for medial compartment loading,[48–50] and the amount of varus thrust.[51] The size of the sustained reduction in the knee adduction moment achieved with HTO deserves emphasis, as it appears to be much larger than reductions achieved when using other biomechanical interventions, such as unloader knee braces or lateral heel wedges.[52,53]

Unfortunately, HTO is a scarcely performed operation compared with other surgical procedures for the degenerative knee.[54] Moreover, data suggest the rates of HTO are decreasing,[55,56] especially in the treatment of knee OA, perhaps because of the small number of surgeons performing the procedure and the limited emphasis in current North American training programs, as well as increased indication for unicompartmental knee arthroplasty. Importantly, HTO is rarely recommended in clinical practice guidelines for knee OA because limited high-level evidence exists to support its inclusion.[57–61] When HTO is incorporated in guidelines, it is generally reserved for more active patients (eg, those with physically demanding jobs) after more advanced joint damage has occurred (defined as medial compartment joint space narrowing, osteophytes, and sclerosis) and conservative interventions have failed.[62]

We agree with the importance of nonoperative interventions shown to improve patients' symptoms as first-line treatments for early knee OA, including degenerative meniscal tears. However, we believe there is strong rationale for also performing realignment surgery before the establishment of definitive radiographic OA. By the time most patients are referred to an orthopedic surgeon for HTO, multiple active biological and physical processes have already been in play and resulted in substantial medial joint damage. We may be waiting too long to intervene with HTO to achieve its greatest benefit. Correcting alignment and thereby lessening aberrant loads on the medial tibiofemoral compartment may be most effective in altering joint disease processes before structural changes can be viewed on radiographs.

It is unfortunate that many of the patients who seek potential surgical treatment options, in addition to nonoperative care, are generally offered arthroscopic meniscectomy and/or debridement without any consideration for realignment surgery. Other patients may be told to persist with nonoperative treatment until their symptoms and radiographic OA severity have progressed enough to be considered candidates for early joint replacement surgery. We believe those treatment strategies represent missed opportunities for potential secondary prevention achieved with HTO.

CLINICAL CASES
Case 1

A 30-year-old male computer programmer was seen in clinic with a history of consistent bilateral medial knee pain over a 5-year period. The patient was quite physically active, having previously played collegiate hockey and national-level baseball. Varus alignment was confirmed for both knees through full-standing hip-to-ankle radiographs, seen in **Fig. 1**A. An MRI of the patient's right knee also confirmed an increased signal of the meniscus, suggesting meniscal degeneration. Therefore, the patient was deemed a suitable candidate for HTO. The patient underwent bilateral HTOs with arthroscopy at a 1-year interval between procedures. Arthroscopy confirmed the presence of a small DMMT during both procedures, which were subsequently resected (**Fig. 1**B, right knee). At 12 years following the second HTO, the patient continued to show good alignment with no evidence of medial compartment damage in either knee joint (see **Fig. 1**A). The patient then suffered a twisting mechanism injury that resulted in a lateral meniscal injury to the right knee. A lateral meniscal repair was

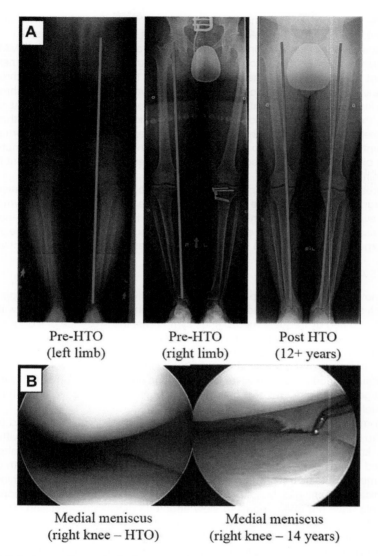

Fig. 1. (*A*) Patient radiographs before and after bilateral HTO surgery. An estimate of the limb weight distribution through the knee is shown with the vertical red line. (*B*) Arthroscopic view of the medial meniscus during HTO and arthroscopy and 14 years after the initial surgery.

then performed on the patient, and it was confirmed that there was still no evidence of further medial meniscal damage 14 years after the initial HTO.

Case 2

A 40-year-old male lawyer and high-performance triathlete was seen in clinic with a 3-year history of persistent bilateral medial compartment pain with physical activity and joint effusion. Three years prior, the patient had undergone a medial arthroscopic partial meniscectomy of the right knee at a different tertiary care center. A full-standing hip-to-ankle radiograph (**Fig. 2**A) showed the patient had definitive varus alignment in both limbs. On physical examination, the patient was diagnosed with a DMMT and subsequently was deemed a candidate for HTO surgery with varus alignment and persistent knee symptoms. The patient underwent bilateral HTOs with arthroscopy at a 1-year interval between procedures. A DMMT was confirmed during arthroscopy for both knees with relatively intact articular cartilage (**Fig. 2**B, right knee). As seen in **Fig. 2**A, the patient did not undergo noticeable radiographic changes in either knee from baseline to 1 year after the second HTO (2 years after first HTO). Fortunately, the patient was able to return to full activities, including rigorous activity (ie, triathlons), after his bilateral HTOs with resolution of his persistent knee pain and without indication of joint effusion.

The presented case studies provide anecdotal proof of principle that a patient with varus alignment and early knee OA (ie, degenerative meniscal tear, knee symptoms, and no evidence of radiographic OA) can undergo HTO and show little-to-no signs of progressed medial meniscal degeneration or radiographic OA even at 12 years after initial surgery, as well as go on to return to preoperative level of rigorous activity.

CAVEATS AND CHALLENGES

We acknowledge that we are, perhaps controversially, suggesting a more aggressive approach than the current standard of care for treating a subset of patients with early knee OA, defined by frequent medial knee symptoms, the presence of a degenerative meniscal tear, and varus alignment. HTO realignment surgery should not be offered by surgeons in a cavalier manner nor be taken lightly by patients who need to be fully informed of its risk and benefits. It is an invasive procedure that involves a prolonged rehabilitation period (ie, progressive weight bearing on crutches) compared with some other surgeries and has a number of well-known potential complications (eg, hardware failure, delayed union, nonunion, loss of correction).

Randomized trials have led to changes in clinical practice guidelines and funding models to limit arthroscopic meniscectomy and/or debridement in patients with radiographic knee OA. However, increasing rates of knee arthroscopy use show the continued willingness of surgeons to perform the procedure on patients with degenerative meniscal tear, despite having been repeatedly shown to provide minimal, if any clinically meaningful benefit, especially long-term. Also, current nonoperative treatments have not been shown to slow structural disease progression. There is a dire need for additional options that can alter the rate of knee joint degeneration.

Unfortunately, decreasing rates of HTO suggest an inability or reluctance of surgeons to perform the procedure or a lack of HTO surgical procedure training. In fact, most orthopedic residents receive little or no experience with HTO during their training, leaving techniques to be learned during fellowships or other continuing medical education courses. To warrant further training, stronger evidence (eg, randomized controlled trials) to support to use of HTO is required.

ADVANCEMENTS IN HIGH TIBIAL OSTEOTOMY TECHNIQUE

Improvements in HTO plate technology and surgical technique have resulted in faster return to weight bearing after surgery[63] and fewer complications[64] than previously reported. For example, development of locking plate designs for osteotomy fixation has allowed patients to begin progressive weight bearing as early as 2 weeks after surgery,[65] much sooner than previous nonlocking plate designs which required a much longer period of non–weight bearing.[66] In addition, studies from orthopedic centers

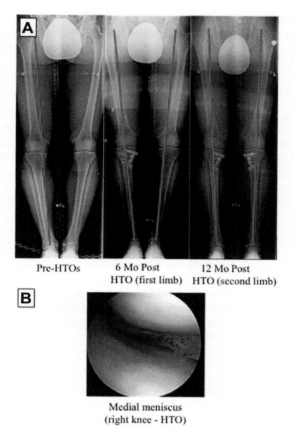

Pre-HTOs   6 Mo Post   12 Mo Post
                  HTO (first limb)   HTO (second limb)

Medial meniscus
(right knee - HTO)

Fig. 2. (*A*) Patient radiographs before and after bilateral HTO surgery. An estimate of the limb weight distribution through the knee is shown with the vertical red line. (*B*) Arthroscopic view of the medial meniscus during HTO.

that perform high volumes of HTO surgery annually have reported complication rates as low as 7%.[64] Moreover, correcting alignment earlier in the disease process in patients who tend to be younger, with less acquired varus and less comorbidities, may enable smaller corrections, faster rehabilitation and fewer complications.

Comparatively, anterior cruciate ligament (ACL) reconstruction and total knee arthroplasty (TKA) are performed very frequently; more than 100,000 per year[67,68] and 1,000,000 per year,[69] respectively, in the United States alone. Studies have reported periods of recovery as long as 6 to 12 months for ACL reconstruction,[70] often longer than rates reported for HTO. Although return to weight bearing is generally faster after TKA, reported complication rates are much higher with TKA[71,72] and TKA places a number of other functional limitations on patients (eg, activity limitations). Still, surgeons continue to perform these surgeries on patients in high volumes to improve symptoms and joint stability. Furthermore, the goals of HTO may vary among surgeons and for specific patient characteristics. We have observed considerable success in improving gait biomechanics and clinical outcomes by correcting alignment to approximately neutral, rather than overcorrecting into substantial valgus.[20,50,73] Yet, despite the reported clinical benefits of HTO and comparable risks to other procedures, the volume of HTO procedures performed annually continues to decline, likely as a result of limited high-quality evidence and a lack of surgeons trained to perform HTO.

FUTURE RESEARCH

We acknowledge that this article provides the lowest form of evidence.[74] Our goal is rather to stimulate discussion and encourage research. Currently, no studies have explored the potential role of realignment surgery for symptomatic patients early in the OA disease process (eg, with degenerative meniscal tear and no radiographic knee OA). We suggest that combined interventions that target individualized risk factors for knee OA progression, including varus alignment, need to be studied and that patients presenting with degenerative meniscal tears are appropriate participants for such studies.

SUMMARY

We propose that HTO is not currently being used to its full potential and warrants future research. The procedure may be particularly useful in patients with recurrent symptoms, varus alignment, and a DMMT, before radiographic damage is evident. HTO in patients with degenerative meniscal tear may present an excellent opportunity for early intervention in patients with varus alignment and symptomatic early knee OA for secondary prevention of radiographic knee OA.

REFERENCES

1. Atukorala I, Kwoh CK, Guermazi A, et al. Synovitis in knee osteoarthritis: a precursor of disease? Ann Rheum Dis 2016;75(2):390–5.

2. Beaufils P, Becker R, Kopf S, et al. The knee meniscus: management of traumatic tears and degenerative lesions. EFORT Open Rev 2017;2(5):195–203.

3. MacFarlane LA, Yang H, Collins JE, et al. Association of changes in effusion-synovitis and progression of cartilage damage over 18 months in patients with osteoarthritis and meniscal tear. Arthritis Rheumatol 2018;71(1): 73–81.

4. Sharma L, Eckstein F, Song J, et al. Relationship of meniscal damage, meniscal extrusion, malalignment, and joint laxity to subsequent cartilage loss in osteoarthritic knees. Arthritis Rheum 2008;58(6):1716–26.

5. Sharma L, Chmiel JS, Almagor O, et al. The role of varus and valgus alignment in the initial development of knee cartilage damage by MRI: the MOST study. Ann Rheum Dis 2013;72(2):235–40.

6. Englund M, Felson DT, Guermazi A, et al. Risk factors for medial meniscal pathology on knee MRI in older US adults: a multicentre prospective cohort study. Ann Rheum Dis 2011;70(10):1733–9.

7. Cicuttini F, Wluka A, Hankin J, et al. Longitudinal study of the relationship between knee angle and tibiofemoral cartilage volume in subjects with knee osteoarthritis. Rheumatology (Oxford) 2004;43(3):321–4.

8. Brouwer GM, van Tol AW, Bergink AP, et al. Association between valgus and varus alignment and the development and progression of radiographic osteoarthritis of the knee. Arthritis Rheum 2007;56(4):1204–11.

9. Cerejo R, Dunlop DD, Cahue S, et al. The influence of alignment on risk of knee osteoarthritis progression according to baseline stage of disease. Arthritis Rheum 2002;46(10):2632–6.

10. Sharma L, Song J, Felson DT, et al. The role of knee alignment in disease progression and functional decline in knee OA. JAMA 2001;286(2):188–95.

11. Sharma L, Song J, Dunlop D, et al. Varus and valgus alignment and incident and progressive knee osteoarthritis. Ann Rheum Dis 2010;69(11):1940–5.

12. Englund M, Guermazi A, Gale D, et al. Incidental meniscal findings on knee MRI in middle-aged and elderly persons. N Engl J Med 2008;359(11):1108–15.

13. Niu J, Felson DT, Neogi T, et al. Patterns of coexisting lesions detected on magnetic resonance imaging and relationship to incident knee osteoarthritis: the multicenter osteoarthritis study. Arthritis Rheumatol 2015;67(12):3158–65.

14. Emmanuel K, Quinn E, Niu J, et al. Quantitative measures of meniscus extrusion predict incident radiographic knee osteoarthritis–data from the osteoarthritis initiative. Osteoarthritis Cartilage 2016;24(2):262–9.

15. Roemer FW, Kwoh CK, Hannon MJ, et al. What comes first? Multitissue involvement leading to radiographic osteoarthritis: magnetic resonance imaging-based trajectory analysis over four years in the osteoarthritis initiative. Arthritis Rheumatol 2015;67(8):2085–96.

16. Sharma L, Nevitt M, Hochberg M, et al. Clinical significance of worsening versus stable preradiographic MRI lesions in a cohort study of persons at higher risk for knee osteoarthritis. Ann Rheum Dis 2016;75(9):1630–6.

17. Teichtahl AJ, Cicuttini FM, Abram F, et al. Meniscal extrusion and bone marrow lesions are associated with incident and progressive knee osteoarthritis. Osteoarthritis Cartilage 2017;25(7):1076–83.

18. Englund M, Guermazi A, Roemer FW, et al. Meniscal tear in knees without surgery and the development of radiographic osteoarthritis among middle-aged and elderly persons: the Multicenter Osteoarthritis Study. Arthritis Rheum 2009; 60(3):831–9.

19. Halder A, Kutzner I, Graichen F, et al. Influence of limb alignment on mediolateral loading in total knee replacement: in vivo measurements in five patients. J Bone Joint Surg Am 2012;94(11):1023–9.

20. Leitch KM, Birmingham TB, Dunning CE, et al. Changes in valgus and varus alignment neutralize aberrant frontal plane knee moments in patients with unicompartmental knee osteoarthritis. J Biomech 2013;46(7):1408–12.

21. Andriacchi TP. Dynamics of knee malalignment. Orthop Clin North Am 1994; 25(3):395–403.

22. Kutzner I, Trepczynski A, Heller MO, et al. Knee adduction moment and medial contact force–facts about their correlation during gait. PLoS One 2013;8(12): e81036.

23. Bennell KL, Bowles KA, Wang Y, et al. Higher dynamic medial knee load predicts greater cartilage loss over 12 months in medial knee osteoarthritis. Ann Rheum Dis 2011;70(10):1770–4.

24. Chang AH, Moisio KC, Chmiel JS, et al. External knee adduction and flexion moments during gait and medial tibiofemoral disease progression in knee osteoarthritis. Osteoarthritis Cartilage 2015;23(7):1099–106.

25. Chehab EF, Favre J, Erhart-Hledik JC, et al. Baseline knee adduction and flexion moments during walking are both associated with 5 year cartilage changes in patients with medial knee osteoarthritis. Osteoarthritis Cartilage 2014;22(11): 1833–9.

26. Miyazaki T, Wada M, Kawahara H, et al. Dynamic load at baseline can predict radiographic disease progression in medial compartment knee osteoarthritis. Ann Rheum Dis 2002;61(7):617–22.

27. Chang A, Hayes K, Dunlop D, et al. Thrust during ambulation and the progression of knee osteoarthritis. Arthritis Rheum 2004;50(12):3897–903.

28. Sharma L, Chang AH, Jackson RD, et al. Varus thrust and incident and progressive knee osteoarthritis. Arthritis Rheumatol 2017;69(11):2136–43.

29. Wink AE, Gross KD, Brown CA, et al. Varus thrust during walking and the risk of incident and worsening medial tibiofemoral MRI lesions: the Multicenter Osteoarthritis Study. Osteoarthritis Cartilage 2017;25(6):839–45.

30. McAlindon TE, Bannuru RR, Sullivan MC, et al. OARSI guidelines for the nonsurgical management of knee osteoarthritis. Osteoarthritis Cartilage 2014;22(3):363–88.

31. Parker DA, Scholes C, Neri T. Non-operative treatment options for knee osteoarthritis: current concepts. J ISAKOS 2018;3(5):274–81.

32. Felson DT, Niu J, Neogi T, et al. Synovitis and the risk of knee osteoarthritis: the MOST Study. Osteoarthritis Cartilage 2016;24(3):458–64.

33. Wang X, Blizzard L, Halliday A, et al. Association between MRI-detected knee joint regional effusion-synovitis and structural changes in older adults: a cohort study. Ann Rheum Dis 2016;75(3):519–25.

34. Wang X, Jin X, Han W, et al. Cross-sectional and longitudinal associations between knee joint effusion synovitis and knee pain in older adults. J Rheumatol 2016;43(1):121–30.

35. Abram SGF, Judge A, Beard DJ, et al. Temporal trends and regional variation in the rate of arthroscopic knee surgery in England: analysis of over 1.7 million procedures between 1997 and 2017. Has practice changed in response to new evidence? Br J Sports Med 2018. https://doi.org/10.1136/bjsports-2018-099414.

36. Stahel PF, Wang P, Huftless S, et al. Surgeon practice patterns of arthroscopic partial meniscectomy for degenerative disease in the united states: a measure of low-value care. JAMA Surg 2018;153(5):494–5.

37. Stone JA, Salzler MJ, Parker DA, et al. Degenerative meniscus tears—assimilation of evidence and consensus statements across three continents: state of the art. J ISAKOS 2017;2(2):108–19.

38. Herrlin S, Hallander M, Wange P, et al. Arthroscopic or conservative treatment of degenerative medial meniscal tears: a prospective randomised trial. Knee Surg Sports Traumatol Arthrosc 2007;15(4):393–401.

39. Herrlin SV, Wange PO, Lapidus G, et al. Is arthroscopic surgery beneficial in treating non-traumatic, degenerative medial meniscal tears? A five year follow-up. Knee Surg Sports Traumatol Arthrosc 2013;21(2):358–64.

40. Katz JN, Brophy RH, Chaisson CE, et al. Surgery versus physical therapy for a meniscal tear and osteoarthritis. N Engl J Med 2013;368(18):1675–84.

41. Kirkley A, Birmingham TB, Litchfield RB, et al. A randomized trial of arthroscopic surgery for OA of the knee. N Engl J Med 2008;359(11):1097–107.

42. Moseley JB, O'Malley K, Petersen NJ, et al. A controlled trial of arthroscopic surgery for osteoarthritis of the knee. N Engl J Med 2002;347(2):81–8.

43. van de Graaf VA, Noorduyn JCA, Willigenburg NW, et al. Effect of early surgery vs physical therapy on knee function among patients with nonobstructive meniscal tears: the ESCAPE randomized clinical trial. JAMA 2018;320(13):1328–37.

44. Kise NJ, Risberg MA, Stensrud S, et al. Exercise therapy versus arthroscopic partial meniscectomy for degenerative meniscal tear in middle aged patients: randomised controlled trial with two year follow-up. BMJ 2016;354:i3740.

45. Sihvonen R, Paavola M, Malmivaara A, et al. Arthroscopic partial meniscectomy versus placebo surgery for a degenerative meniscus tear: a 2-year follow-up of the randomised controlled trial. Ann Rheum Dis 2018;77(2):188–95.

46. Sihvonen R, Paavola M, Malmivaara A, et al. Arthroscopic partial meniscectomy versus sham surgery for a degenerative meniscal tear. N Engl J Med 2013; 369(26):2515–24.

47. Yim JH, Seon JK, Song EK, et al. A comparative study of meniscectomy and nonoperative treatment for degenerative horizontal tears of the medial meniscus. Am J Sports Med 2013;41(7):1565–70.

48. Prodromos CC, Andriacchi TP, Galante JO. A relationship between gait and clinical changes following high tibial osteotomy. J Bone Joint Surg Am 1985;67(8): 1188–94.

49. Lind M, McClelland J, Wittwer JE, et al. Gait analysis of walking before and after medial opening wedge high tibial osteotomy. Knee Surg Sports Traumatol Arthrosc 2013;21(1):74–81.

50. Birmingham TB, Moyer R, Leitch K, et al. Changes in biomechanical risk factors for knee osteoarthritis and their association with 5-year clinically important improvement after limb realignment surgery. Osteoarthritis Cartilage 2017; 25(12):1999–2006.

51. Deie M, Hoso T, Shimada N, et al. Differences between opening versus closing high tibial osteotomy on clinical outcomes and gait analysis. Knee 2014;21(6): 1046–51.

52. Moyer R, Birmingham T, Dombroski C, et al. Combined versus individual effects of a valgus knee brace and lateral wedge foot orthotic during stair use in patients with knee osteoarthritis. Gait Posture 2017;54:160–6.

53. Moyer RF, Birmingham TB, Dombroski CE, et al. Combined effects of a valgus knee brace and lateral wedge foot orthotic on the external knee adduction moment in patients with varus gonarthrosis. Arch Phys Med Rehabil 2013; 94(1):103–12.

54. Dhawan A, Mather RC 3rd, Karas V, et al. An epidemiologic analysis of clinical practice guidelines for non-arthroplasty treatment of osteoarthritis of the knee. Arthroscopy 2014;30(1):65–71.

55. W-Dahl A, Robertsson O, Lohmander LS. High tibial osteotomy in Sweden, 1998-2007: a population-based study of the use and rate of revision to knee arthroplasty. Acta Orthop 2012;83(3):244–8.

56. Niinimaki TT, Eskelinen A, Ohtonen P, et al. Incidence of osteotomies around the knee for the treatment of knee osteoarthritis: a 22-year population-based study. Int Orthop 2012;36(7):1399–402.

57. Hochberg MC, Altman RD, April KT, et al. American College of Rheumatology 2012 recommendations for the use of nonpharmacologic and pharmacologic therapies in osteoarthritis of the hand, hip, and knee. Arthritis Care Res 2012; 64(4):465–74.

58. Jevsevar DS. Treatment of osteoarthritis of the knee: evidence-based guideline, 2nd edition. J Am Acad Orthop Surg 2013;21(9):571–6.

59. Scott J, Checketts JX, Horn JG, et al. Knee osteoarthritis and current research for evidence-are we on the right way? Int Orthop 2018;42(9):2105–12.

60. Carlson VR, Ong AC, Orozco FR, et al. Compliance with the AAOS Guidelines for treatment of osteoarthritis of the knee: a survey of the American Association of Hip and Knee Surgeons. J Am Acad Orthop Surg 2018;26(3):103–7.

61. Zhang W, Moskowitz RW, Nuki G, et al. OARSI recommendations for the management of hip and knee osteoarthritis, Part II: OARSI evidence-based, expert consensus guidelines. Osteoarthritis Cartilage 2008;16(2):137–62.

62. Bruyere O, Cooper C, Pelletier JP, et al. An algorithm recommendation for the management of knee osteoarthritis in Europe and internationally: a report from a task force of the European Society for Clinical and Economic Aspects of Osteoporosis and Osteoarthritis (ESCEO). Semin Arthritis Rheum 2014;44(3): 253–63.

63. Lee OS, Ahn S, Lee YS. Effect and safety of early weight-bearing on the outcome after open-wedge high tibial osteotomy: a systematic review and meta-analysis. Arch Orthop Trauma Surg 2017;137(7):903–11.

64. Martin R, Birmingham TB, Willits K, et al. Adverse event rates and classifications in medial opening wedge high tibial osteotomy. Am J Sports Med 2014;42(5): 1118–26.

65. Hernigou P, Queinnec S, Picard L, et al. Safety of a novel high tibial osteotomy locked plate fixation for immediate full weight-bearing: a case-control study. Int Orthop 2013;37(12):2377–84.

66. Asik M, Sen C, Kilic B, et al. High tibial osteotomy with Puddu plate for the treatment of varus gonarthrosis. Knee Surg Sports Traumatol Arthrosc 2006;14(10): 948–54.

67. Buller LT, Best MJ, Baraga MG, et al. Trends in anterior cruciate ligament reconstruction in the United States. Orthop J Sports Med 2015;3(1). 2325967114563664.

68. Mall NA, Chalmers PN, Moric M, et al. Incidence and trends of anterior cruciate ligament reconstruction in the United States. Am J Sports Med 2014;42(10): 2363–70.

69. Inacio MCS, Paxton EW, Graves SE, et al. Projected increase in total knee arthroplasty in the United States - an alternative projection model. Osteoarthritis Cartilage 2017;25(11):1797–803.

70. Adams D, Logerstedt DS, Hunter-Giordano A, et al. Current concepts for anterior cruciate ligament reconstruction: a criterion-based rehabilitation progression. J Orthop Sports Phys Ther 2012;42(7):601–14.

71. Atkinson HDE. The negatives of knee replacement surgery: complications and the dissatisfied patient. Orthopaedics and Trauma 2017;31(1):25–33.

72. Belmont PJ Jr, Goodman GP, Waterman BR, et al. Thirty-day postoperative complications and mortality following total knee arthroplasty: incidence and risk factors among a national sample of 15,321 patients. J Bone Joint Surg Am 2014; 96(1):20–6.

73. Birmingham TB, Giffin JR, Chesworth BM, et al. Medial opening wedge high tibial osteotomy: a prospective cohort study of gait, radiographic, and patient-reported outcomes. Arthritis Rheum 2009;61(5):648–57.

74. Balshem H, Helfand M, Schunemann HJ, et al. GRADE guidelines: 3. Rating the quality of evidence. J Clin Epidemiol 2011;64(4):401–6.

Moving?

Make sure your subscription moves with you!

To notify us of your new address, find your **Clinics Account Number** (located on your mailing label above your name), and contact customer service at:

Email: journalscustomerservice-usa@elsevier.com

800-654-2452 (subscribers in the U.S. & Canada)
314-447-8871 (subscribers outside of the U.S. & Canada)

Fax number: 314-447-8029

Elsevier Health Sciences Division
Subscription Customer Service
3251 Riverport Lane
Maryland Heights, MO 63043

Moving?

Make sure your subscription moves with you!

To notify us of your new address, find your Clinics Account Number (located on your mailing label above your name), and contact customer service at:

Email: JournalsCustomerService-usa@elsevier.com

800-654-2452 (subscribers in the U.S. & Canada)
314-447-8871 (subscribers outside of the U.S. & Canada)

Fax number: 314-447-8029

Elsevier Health Sciences Division
Subscription Customer Service
3251 Riverport Lane
Maryland Heights, MO 63043

To ensure uninterrupted delivery of your subscription, please notify us at least 4 weeks in advance of move.

Printed and bound by CPI Group (UK) Ltd, Croydon, CR0 4YY

08/05/2025

01864745-0009